O.M.G
MY KID IS
OVERWEIGHT

STOP!

I want to give you more.

Claim NOW your

WORKBOOK

FOR FREE

If you have not downloaded the workbook
Yet and you want to get faster results.
Download the workbook now!

How? Easy!

GO TO:

www.omgoverweight.com/WORKBOOK

I'm not sure...

That this offer will stay always for **FREE**... so hurry up

O.M.G My Kid Is OVERWEIGHT

The complete guide for raising physically and emotionally healthy children

© 2018 BAR AIZIK

Visit the author's website at:

www.baraizik.com

Table of Contents

INTRODUCTION

What made me write this book?

I believe that the influence the parent has on the child is huge.

The parent has a number of very significant roles that take a large part in shaping the child's personality and development as a physically healthy and emotionally balanced child.

However, parents today do not always have practical tools to raise healthy and balanced children. This book is brought to you as a theoretical and practical guide to raising healthy children in body and mind.

According to the World Health Organization (WHO), worldwide obesity has nearly tripled since 1975. In 2016, more than 1.9 billion adults, 18 years and older, were overweight. Of these, over 650 million adults were obese. 41 million children under the age of 5 were overweight or obese in 2016.

Over 340 million children and adolescents aged 5-19 were overweight or obese in 2016.

But the most important fact I want you remember is that **obesity is preventable**!

According to health care estimates in 2013, being overweight and obese led to the premature death of 4.5 million people around the world. Of course, health risks increase as the weight gain increases.

Being overweight has many effects on physical and mental health for every child or adult who suffers from this.

People who are overweight or obese have been found to suffer significantly more from diseases like type 1 and type 2 diabetes, arthritis, high blood pressure, cholesterol, and even various cancers. Emotionally, obese people have suffered more from depression, anxiety, loneliness, lack of self-confidence, and more.

The increase in obesity as a social phenomenon stems mainly from changes in diet and patterns of physical activity that have changed greatly in recent years and continue to change. The development of the world leads to the fact that, in many families, both the husband and the wife develop a career parallel to raising their children. This makes it difficult for any prolonged discussion of healthy foods. Today, there is a large variety of fast food and prepared food that significantly shortens the entire process of food preparation. The problem with this is that it is impossible to know exactly what we are putting into our mouths. In addition to the problematic consumer culture that developed, the amount of activity a person performs during the day has dropped significantly compare to people of the past. People use electric bicycles and other ways of transportation and do less physical activity.

Sometimes, it is very difficult to understand what is right and what is not right to do, what is permitted and what is forbidden, what to feed more of and what to feed less of, how long a child should be allowed to play on the computer or not at all, and when to set a limit on something and when to allow it.

I have noticed that many parents are dealing with children who are overweight or obese. There are many questions and unresolved holes in this complex equation, and sometimes it is difficult for a parent to know what the best thing is to do for the good of the child. I have no doubt that every parent wants the best for his children and that each child has his own personality and his special character. But, not every parent knows what is really good for their child. In case you do not see the overall picture of the equation, it can really be that the formula is difficult to crack. But, once you learn all the aspects and begin to see the full picture, you can see how all the pieces form a complete and clear picture.

The holistic formula on which I wrote this book is based on four main components

- Body and mind
- Environment and habits
- Nutrition
- Physical activity

In this book, I will talk about the holistic view of things. The holistic word derives from the word *whole*. This is a broader view of each of the factors, and looks at each person as a whole and not just as a physical body as we usually do. A broader view will allow us to see a number of new angles and ways of thinking to address any issue of being overweight or obese.

This book will help you understand all parts of the equation and see the broad picture. You will receive clear tools to help you deal with all issues of being overweight and raising healthy and balanced children. Every parent wants his child to have all the tools to become a healthy, happy, satisfied, and successful person. Right now, you are holding in your hands a tool that can help you give all these things that you wish for your children.

About the author

My name is Bar Aizik, and I have been a fitness trainer for over ten years now. I started my professional career in high school and received my qualifications as a fitness coach and a children's coach after three years of study. After completing high school, I enlisted in the IDF and served as a fitness trainer and Krav Maga instructor for three years.

During that time, I went to work with thousands of soldiers in different units and helped them get into shape. I continued to specialize in fitness and continued to work as a personal fitness trainer in order to help children and adults improve their quality of life and live healthier lives while reaching their goals.

Parallel to my occupation as a fitness trainer, I studied for four years as a holistic psychotherapist. The knowledge I acquired during my studies helped me to see and understand the overall picture and to make the connection between the human body and mind. I understood there was much more than one shoe in the equation and to make a change, it was necessary to treat the human mind and not just to emphasize the correct sports and nutrition.

In order to fully understand the impact of the environment and the habits on a person, I underwent various training programs. Among them, I was certified as a neuro-linguistic programming (NLP) therapist. It is a method that offers a variety of psychological techniques and skills designed to generate influences and changes in thought, emotions, and behaviors, and, through this change of habits, program patterns and harness them to achieve the desired results.

I developed and wrote this entire book thanks to many years of independent learning and research that began at the age of sixteen. I took everything I learned from different disciplines like sports nutrition, and mind changing habits, and I attached the experience I had accumulated over ten years to one method that touches all aspects and is easy to implement.

The holistic formula

Being overweight or obese has become more prevalent today than ever before. We have come across theories in various methods that try to deal with the same phenomenon worldwide, and this is, undoubtedly, one of the biggest struggles currently in existence. Today, we learn about a healthy way of life in the educational systems, such as schools and television programs. But, although there is more awareness, the situation has not improved, and every year the percentage of obese children increases. If the ads are more common and there is so much publicity about the same problematic issue, how is it possible that the trend is so negative? This question and many more will be answered in this book.

But where did it all start? What causes this obesity and how has it become so widespread in recent years? What is the right approach? How do we know what to choose and which route to take?

My answer to you is very simple. In my opinion, it is not possible to point to just one thing that causes obesity, just as one cannot point to one thing that causes cancer.

Each of the four topics I mentioned earlier can cause a person to become overweight or obese.

A person's mental state contributes if they are feeling anxiety, pressure, and so forth. Their habits and physical environment may not have supported a healthy lifestyle. They may be suffering from poor nutrition or a lack of physical activity. The problem is that many authority figures look at obesity issues from one point of view according to their world view and according to their field of activity.

For example, nutritionists say it's a matter of nutrition, fitness coaches say obesity is due to a lack of physical activity, and psychologists say it is due to emotional eating. There is not one approach that is the most correct, and all these approaches have a significant part in the process of change. One of the four parts is very important and each part has an impact on another. Once you look at the same subject only through one angle, the picture will never be complete. For example, a person who suffers from emotional eating, if he only takes care of his diet, he will not be able to lose weight and maintain it for long, because any crisis or mental difficulty he experiences will return him to the starting point, and he does not have the necessary tools to cope with the situation.

Most people return to their starting weight after trying a weight loss process, because the source of the problem was not resolved. If we take the same person and, instead, send him to a nutritionist and to a psychologist and work on the emotional pressures and traumas that are probably causing his obesity, we can see how slowly he will begin to understand why he is in this situation. He will internalize where the problems come from and his compulsive eating will fade slowly and his nutrition will be more controlled and balanced.

Of course, once a person has started to see results, the positive trend is going to get easier, and he will stick to the proper diet and healthier lifestyle so that he can continue to enjoy the results. When a person has all the tools needed to fully assimilate the meaning of a long and healthy life, this understanding will allow him to make a profound change in his thinking, and he will be able to maintain this change over time.

We talked about the holistic view of the subject of obesity at the beginning of the book. Now let's go over it a bit more and understand more deeply each of the four sections.

Body and mind

There are many studies that prove that the state of mind affects the body. This is a very complex issue, and we are far from understanding it all. What the same approach says is that there are many situations in our lives—for example, as a result of mental stress, crisis, trauma, or tragedy that a person experiences—which can lead a person to an increased consumption of food to compensate for the painful issues experienced by their mind.

This situation I describe here—and you probably recognize the concept—is known as "emotional eating." Emotional eating is defined as "an increase in food consumption in response to negative emotions" and is considered an adaptive coping method to severe emotions. Although emotional eating is not listed in the American Psychiatric Association's Diagnostic and

Statistical Manual, it is considered a type of eating disorder and is treated accordingly. This means that the source of compulsive eating and obesity is not necessarily the result of a poor diet itself, but the effect of the internal state of the human psyche that leads to increased consumption of these foods in order to cope with different situations.

Environment and habits

There are studies that show the great impact your environment has on your habits. This means that if a person is born into a family that is athletic and healthy, there is a high chance that they will grow up as a healthy child and that sport will be part of their lifestyle. Conversely, if a person is born into a family that is not active and does not eat healthily, it is more likely that the same child will become obese, even if they did not suffer from obesity in the early years of their childhood. The question that develops around this approach is why we see more and more families where the parents are a normal weight while one or more of their children are overweight or obese.

Nutrition

Many factors point an accusing finger at our consumer culture and fast-food chains that allow, today more than ever, everyone to get very tasty and cheap food. Another fact is that today people consume more food away from home than food in the home. In many families, both parents are developing a career in parallel with raising children, which makes it difficult for time and attention to be given to the whole issue of nutrition, and we turn to more rapid alternatives and availability. In addition, there is the wonder of the food chains. Many times junk food is disguised as a healthy food: diet cola, cereals made from five types of cereals, etc. The food industry knows what we are looking for and knows exactly what to display to attract buyers. On the one hand, customers want to buy healthier foods, but, on the other hand, how can they really do this with all the advertising delusions and distractions that surround foods. The question is can we really know what is healthy and what is not when the goal of those huge organizations is to sell us more and more?

Physical activity

Some experts say that the problem is that there is no physical activity, that everything has become so accessible that it is easy to get anywhere easily and effortlessly with electric bicycles, electric scooters, cars, etc. Technological advances (with all its goodwill), on the one hand, help us in so many ways, from transportation to medicine, but on the other hand, make everyone less and less active. Over the years, people find themselves less and less active and spend their free time in front of television screens, computer screens, and telephone screens.

Being overweight in the modern world

Before we begin to go into the depth of things and go through each step, it is important to understand the order of things. I have concentrated the basic knowledge that is important to know about obesity and its effects, and, after you understand the background, you will be clearer on other parts of the book.

Consequences of being overweight or obese

What is metabolic syndrome?

The metabolic syndrome is accumulated symptoms that increase the risk of type 2 diabetes or cardiovascular disease. Its characteristics are abdominal obesity, high blood pressure, high blood triglyceride levels or low levels of HDL in the blood, and fasting hyperglycemia. The syndrome is also known as X syndrome or insulin resistance syndrome, and, when combined, they increase the risk of type 2 diabetes or cardiovascular disease.

According to the ATP3 study, in order to diagnose metabolic syndrome, there is no need for all but three criteria to appear. In Europe, two criteria are sufficient, along with abdominal obesity. The main criteria included in the syndrome are

- Hypertension
- High levels of triglycerides in the blood
- Low levels of HDL in the blood
- Hypoglycemia in fasting

Being overweight or obese are health risk factors for several major non-communicable diseases that are becoming more and more common in children. In the past, these were diseases that were seen mostly in adults.

Here are some of them
- Heart disease and stroke
- Diabetes type 1, and 2
- Osteoarthritis
- several cancer types

Consequences of childhood obesity

According to an article that was published in the *New England Journal of Medicine* (Childhood Adiposity, Adult Adiposity, and Cardiovascular Risk Factors–2011), 82% of children who were obese in childhood continued to suffer from obesity in adulthood.

The research looked at four studies conducted in the United States, Finland, and Australia with 6,328 patients, with an average age of 11.4 years. The research lasted about 23 years.

Subjects were divided into four groups: (1) thin adults who were thin children, (2) thin adults who were obese children, (3) obese adults who were obese children, and (4) obese adults who were thin children. Fatty adults who were obese as a child were 5.4 times more likely to develop type 2 diabetes than adults who maintained a normal weight throughout their lives. In addition, people who were obese throughout life had a 2.7-fold increased risk of developing hypertension, a 1.8-fold increased risk of LDL (bad cholesterol), a 2.1-fold higher risk of HDL ("good" cholesterol), a 3-fold increased risk of increased triglyceride levels, and a 1.7-fold higher risk of developing atherosclerosis.

People who were fat in adulthood, but were thin as children, were able to avoid the increased risk of disease. Among normal-weight adults who were obese children, the risks were the same as those who were never obese. This study highlights the importance of early intervention in the treatment of childhood obesity.

Implications for the emotional state of being overweight

From the first grade, children begin to compare themselves to other children. Once the child sees himself as different, or others behave differently toward him because of his weight, this can lead to sensitive problems and social rejection.

Here are some of the consequences that overweight children suffer from

Low self-esteem

As we have mentioned, children are not always the nicest. A child who suffers from being overweight suffers from a much more unpleasant attitude and discomfort than a child who is a normal weight. In addition to this, the media mainly promotes models and thin actors that appear everywhere and that can cause a decline in the self-confidence of the child. All of this can lead to social isolation and a higher probability of mental states such as depression.

Behavior problems and academic difficulties
Children who are overweight are more likely to suffer from anxiety and social difficulties. These can cause behavioral problems at school, and stress and anxiety can also impair the ability to concentrate and learn.

Depression
Social isolation and low self-esteem can create a feeling of helplessness and hopelessness in children who are overweight. A depressed child may lose interest in ordinary activities that are typical of children his age, they may want to sleep more than usual, and they may cry more. Depression is a serious concern for children and adolescents.

Who is considered overweight or obese?

There are several ways to check to see if a child or adult is overweight or obese. There are devices that test fat with electrical conductivity. A caliper is a pincher that helps measure body fat percentage, and more professional instruments, whose testing is done in a pond, are called hydrostatic body fat testers. There are several ways to check if a person is in a proper weight and fat range. The most judgmental and most popular way to test this is with the help of a BMI Table and a body mass index. The BMI index helps us see whether that person is in the normal range or overweight or obese This table can give you an idea of where your children are standing without having to do special tests.

So, what is body mass index (BMI)?

It is a measure that gives a quantitative assessment of whether a person is in a normal weight, overweight, or underweight range. The index is calculated using height and weight data.

In this chapter, you will find a table that shows where you and your children are in the table, which will give you an indication of where you are and what your situation is in terms of BMI.

So, what is the proper weight?

- A BMI below 18.5 is underweight
- The normal weight of people ranges from BMI values of 18.5 to 25.
- A BMI value over 25 is known as overweight.
- A BMI above 30 is called obesity.
- A BMI index over 40 is called morbid obesity and that is an even more extreme state.

The disadvantage of this measure is that it refers only to your height and does not take into account the width of the human skeleton as well as the lack of reference to the distribution of fat in the body and the lack of separation between the various body components—fat and muscle.

For example, people who exercise in the gym and develop massive muscle tissue, instead of fat tissue, will still weigh more. In this case, for example, the percentage of fat in their bodies is very low, but they may remain in the same BMI percentile because the table does not separate the components of the same weight (in this case muscle).

A well-known example of the BMI's inaccuracy is Michael Jordan, who at the height of his physical fitness had BMI values of 27-29, which are considered being overweight. Although the percentage of fat was very low, the values were the result of his high muscle mass and structure. Still, for what we need, it can be enough for a start and, if necessary, turn on a red light for us to see if there is a negative trend.

BMI for children

As with adults, overweight children are usually measured using the body mass index (BMI). But, in contrast to adult BMI scores in which each outcome enters pre-determined ranges, in children and adolescents, being overweight is defined as a BMI score above 85 percent for their age and sex. An obese child is defined as having a BMI score above 95 percent and underweight is defined as a BMI score below 5 percent for their age and sex.

Is fat necessary or dangerous?

Despite all we know about obesity and the many effects it has, remember that fat is not the enemy. Fat is essential to our survival. A healthy body requires a minimum amount of fat for the functioning of different systems such as

- Hormonal system
- Immune system
- Thermal insulation
- Protection from shocks to sensitive organs
- Energy storage

BMI charts

2 to 20 years: Boys
Stature-for-age and Weight-for-age percentiles

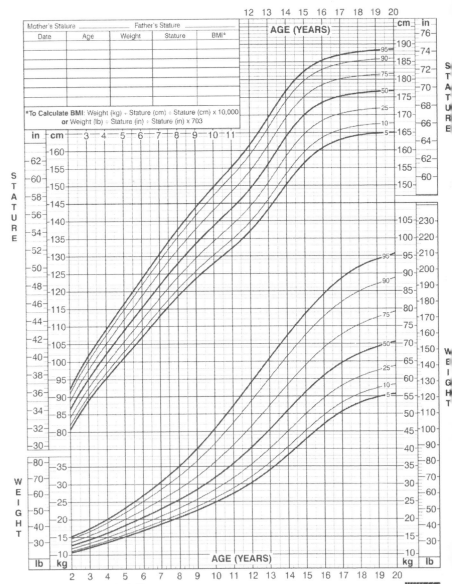

Mother's Stature _____ Father's Stature _____

Date	Age	Weight	Stature	BMI*

*To Calculate BMI: Weight (kg) ÷ Stature (cm) ÷ Stature (cm) x 10,000
or Weight (lb) ÷ Stature (in) ÷ Stature (in) x 703

AGE (YEARS)

STATURE

WEIGHT

Published May 30, 2000 (modified 11/21/00).
SOURCE: Developed by the National Center for Health Statistics in collaboration with
the National Center for Chronic Disease Prevention and Health Promotion (2000).
http://www.cdc.gov/growthcharts

CDC

SAFER · HEALTHIER · PEOPLE"

2 to 20 years: Girls
Stature-for-age and Weight-for-age percentiles

NAME

RECORD #

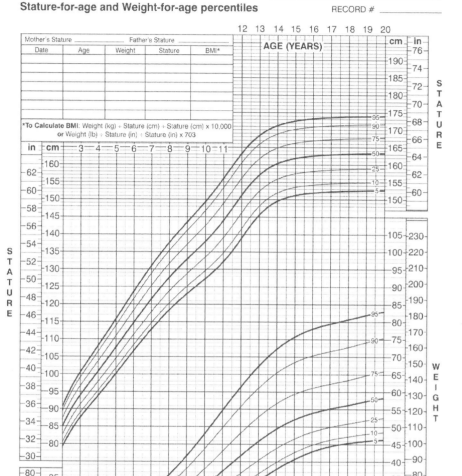

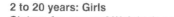

Published May 30, 2000 (modified 11/21/00).
SOURCE: Developed by the National Center for Health Statistics in collaboration with
the National Center for Chronic Disease Prevention and Health Promotion (2000).
http://www.cdc.gov/growthcharts

SAFER • HEALTHIER • PEOPLE

The struggles of an overweight child

Being a fat child in today's society is not pleasant. At a very young age, the child will not notice the difference between himself and his friends, but as the years pass and the children develop and grow, they begin to compare themselves to their environment. This process happens around the age of 6, when an overweight child is naturally exposed to comments and criticisms from his classmates. Children are children, and they do not think twice before saying something.

One of the least pleasant things that can happen to a child is being laughed at in class and called names because he is defined as "different." The unpleasant experience that the child has to go through can be prevented in most cases. If you are at the height of the same situation, I want to tell you to take a deep breath, as it is going to be a long journey. Like you, many people have helped their overweight children reach a normal weight. It is important that you realize that it is entirely possible, as someone has already managed to do it, without having these special links. Simply by following the application of these simple steps, you can help your children to live healthier and more balanced lives.

Is it okay to be fat?

A new aspect is created around every issue of being overweight around the world on the part of those people who come to show and prove that it is okay to be obese, as no one is born perfect, and we should love ourselves as we are. I agree with every word, and I really think that everyone should accept themselves as they are. I think the purpose of those people is truly amazing. Everyone deserves to love himself and see all the good things that exist in him, and everyone deserves to be loved and accepted as they are.

This all sounds good, but let's see you explain it to a child suffering from endless harassment in school. A child suffers from bullying because he is a little different. A heavy child just wants to enjoy and play like everyone else. This innocent child will not be able to understand what you are trying to tell him at such a young age. He will not understand that he is special and there are so many good things in him.

And you cannot educate all the children to accept the obese child in one day. I wish it were so simple. With all the good will there is, it is not really possible to change what society and children think about being overweight and obesity. It should also be remembered that beyond the path to educate the child, the media dictates to us what is right, what is wrong, what is considered different, and what is considered the norm. Children see television characters actors and models as the ideal thing. Media creates a situation where what is different is not acceptable.

In the vast majority of cases, the characters in the television shows and movies are thin people and that makes us consider it the ideal weight. If you live in Japan and you are a sumo wrestler, the public will admire you; the bigger the sumo wrestler, the more attractive they are. But, as we do not live in Japan and we are not sumo wrestlers, it is less relevant. I don't think everyone should have a flat stomach, but I think everyone should be healthy and love his or her body. And, as we have understood so far, obesity and morbid obesity directly relate to the health and mental state of the person.

I love myself as I am

I think you should love yourself in any situation, even if you have 120 extra pounds. But, on the other hand, it is important to understand that there is no connection between self-love and neglect of the body. I have met people who say that they are 100 pounds more than they should be, but they love themselves as they are. I am very happy to hear about the fact that a person really loves himself and accepts himself as he is. But, once it reaches the point that it harms the person's health, performing simple tasks like climbing the stairs or even getting out of bed could be accompanied by chronic fatigue and other effects. And, their blood tests will not be good, and their overall health will be poor. Maybe that person really loves himself just as he is, and that's amazing, and it's important. But, if his body does not like the situation he is in, it affects his health, and that is a completely different story.

"Take care of your body. It's the only place you have to live." - Jim Rohn

---

32

What do children think about obesity?

A new study of four-year-olds found that most of them had already learned to develop a social aversion to obesity, and even characterized obese people as unhappy and unsuccessful. Although most children at this age do not even know how to read, it has been discovered that children of this age know how to do something unusual that, until now, has been thought of as something that only adults do—to discriminate on the basis of external appearance. A study among preschoolers found that most of them had already learned to develop an aversion to obesity. Unfortunately, that shows us how much the aversion to obesity begins at such young ages.

The study was conducted at the University of Leeds in London with 126 boys and girls aged 4. One study presented the children with the same cartoon characters named after "Alfie," but each one had a different characteristic. In this case, there was one normal character, one fat character, and one disabled character in a wheelchair, and the children were asked with whom they would like to play. The fat character was always chosen last, time after time. The children always preferred the normal cartoon character, and then the disabled character, before choosing the fat character.

A story told to the children by the head of the study, Professor Andrew Hill, described a group of children whose naughty cat was stuck on a tall tree and could not get off. Each time the story was told, the main character was replaced by another version of Alfie, and the children were asked to give an opinion. The children agreed that obese Alfie's chances to save the cat were low. The disabled Alfie received more points, and most children chose the normal Alfie. Only a few children said they would like to be a friend of the obese Alfie (only three percent). The experiment was also performed on a female version of Alfie, and the results were the same.

When should we start?

As to when, the answer is very simple - you should start now! If you teach those habits and the way of life at a very young age, the easier it will be for your children much later. Why? There are two main reasons.

Mentally

The younger the child, the easier it is to teach them. Think about it for a moment. Think how easily children learn things. You've heard the concept that a child's brain is like a sponge, and that's right.

A "young age" means that the brain is not yet established and has not yet reached its final shape. It changes and develops according to what it goes through during life. During life, connections are created in the brain. These connections cause us to act or behave in a certain way. For that matter, a young child who played with a dog and got bitten can grow and develop and become an adult with a fear of dogs. That person has created a connection between danger and a fear of dogs and, therefore, every time he sees a dog, he will be afraid. If that person grows up and decides that he wants to get rid of that anxiety, he will have to work much harder because that connection has been established in his brain.

The opposite is to take a parent who had the tools and knew how to deal with the anxiety that the child experienced following the dog's assault. That same parent will help the child to gradually overcome the trauma experienced by the dog, and the parent will show the child that not all dogs are like that. The child will probably not remember the traumatic event, whereas the child who received no help remains traumatized for life. The younger the child begins, the more he will enjoy the benefits of healthy and correct habits and the right to live a healthy life.

Physiologically
As the years pass, it will be more difficult for a child to return to a healthy and proper weight.

One of the reasons is that the body produces mainly fat cells up to the age of 20. If the child is obese, the body will produce fat cells, because the body thinks it needs them. Fat cells in the body will not be able to disappear. The statement of *fat burning* is not that accurate, because you cannot get rid of those fat cells. What happens is that those fat cells shrink. The fat cells have the ability to shrink and expand like a sponge. A large amount of fat cells can lead to a permanent increase in weight gain in the future. In addition to this, there is also a hormonal injury, as obesity has a great impact on the human body. Obesity harms our ability to stabilize the level of sugar in our blood that takes an important part in weight loss.

If they did not make a change at a young age, it can hurt a child into old age and cause him mental scars as he wars with his body image and weight. For example, people who fight for years with their weight cannot give up the things they love so much. They lose dozens of pounds and, after a short time, go back to their previous diet and gain much more.

So what do we understand from that?

The younger you start, the more likely you are to have a child who loves himself, has self-confidence, and lives a healthy life. In addition, the child can enjoy the whole process, because children love to learn. It does not have to be an experience like *The Biggest Loser*. It can be an enjoyable process, as the whole family goes through it together. During the same family change, the parent will have the opportunity to teach the children to make the right choices in terms of nutrition, like what foods to eat and what foods to avoid. The child will have the opportunity to experience different foods. The child will enjoy the consolidation, and they will enjoy the gradual progression of family relationships.

Is surgery the ultimate solution?

Why should we have to endure the whole process of losing weight and building these habits if surgery can be done to solve all these headaches?

Let's talk about what weight loss surgeries include.

There are several types of surgeries that help obese people to lose weight. There is gastric bypass surgery, gastric tightening with rings or staples, and many more. Although the percentage of complications is relatively low, over the years, medicine has progressed and further reduces the risk of these surgeries. But, there are still risks, such as the more dangerous stomach leaks, pulmonary embolisms, internal bleeding, recurrent vomiting, gallstones, and kidney stones.

But the most common problem is that the nutritional deficiencies are extensive and particularly significant in gastric bypass surgery and duodenal bypass, based on reduced absorption. It also occurs in ring surgeries and gastric sleeve surgeries, which are based on reducing the size of the stomach. A lack of nutrients may cause additional complications, such as various neurological disorders and, sometimes, paralysis. Other complications that may occur are osteoporosis and osteopenia, and an increased risk of cardiovascular disease.

Who can have the surgery?

- For most surgeries, the person should be above the BMI 40 index, which is considered morbidly obese.
- In many cases, people who have a BMI of 35 are also admitted to surgery if they suffer from one or more obesity complications such as high blood pressure, heart disease, apnea, fatty liver, etc.
- And there are other cases where the operation is required for people under the age of 35.

Is it worth it or not to have the surgery?

In most cases, it is possible to solve the obesity problem without surgical intervention. But, with the right process and with the appropriate and professional accompaniment, there are some extreme cases that do not allow any other option. It is very important to understand that the surgery itself may change the feeling of hunger and the ability to eat a large amount of food, but if there is no change in their way of thinking and behavior, the person's perception of nutrition will not change. He will continue to behave and think *obese* and go back to his initial weight.

Why is this happening in many cases? Eating under these circumstances is emotional eating without any deep treatment for the mind. The solution of surgery will be superficial, and it will last for a short period until they return to the same habits that they had been accustomed to.

In the event that there is no alternative, and this is the only solution, the only way that the operation will last for a long period of time is through professional help, which will include professional therapy and guidance to change dietary habits and everything needed to make the transition as correctly as possible.

Following many of these surgeries, the same people who did the operation and did not work on the mental part of the whole issue find a way to "bypass" the idea of completing the emotional deprivation that has not yet been solved. They can do it with the aid of putting high-calorie shakes in their hands, grinding chocolates and cookies so finely that they will pass through as a drink so they will be less affected by the rapid feeling of satiety created by the surgery. In the chapters on the body and mind and the environment and habits, I speak more deeply about every part of emotional eating and what things can be done in order to work on those parts that will bring a long-term change.

Consultation and professional assistance

It seems that too often, "shame" plays a role with parents. They feel that their child does not need help, they repress the obvious, and create a situation in which "everything is okay with my child." They think that they can handle any situation on their own, and this creates a situation where the treatment is avoided that could have helped the child overcome the distress at an early stage. The repression of the problem does not solve it, and it certainly doesn't help the child. If you have trouble making changes or do not know what to do or if this is true for your child, you can always consult a doctor. The doctor can see whether this is an initial obesity problem or whether it is a medical problem. The doctor identifies the problem with his experience and a variety of evaluation tools.

Come on, let's start with new beginnings and new actions on the way to a new life

CHAPTER 1: WHAT IS YOUR "WHY"?

The first step

You made the first step and decided to read this book. The title of the book is clear and you already know what it is about but, first of all, I want you to ask yourself the next question: what is the reason you decided to read this book? What motivated you to start reading this book *now*? Maybe it's for the accumulation of knowledge or you have a child in an overweight home and you turned to this book to know more about this topic.

If you read this book, you are concerned about and love the people who are close to you. You want to help your children live a healthier life and live a good quality of life. Anyone who reads this book can bring about a significant change in their children's personal lives by following the same simple and straightforward steps as are described in this book.

Although all this knowledge is in your possession, and even though you know and believe that the material written in this book can help you change the life of your family, only a small portion of those who hold this book will read the whole book to the end and apply everything written in it (usually, the percentage is twenty percent).

You're probably wondering what happened to the rest of the people. Some will not finish the book and many will not be willing to do what is needed to change the life of their family from one end to the other. The big question is what distinguishes those people who made the change and those who did not make the change. In the beginning, everyone's goal was more or less the same.

That's what I'm going to talk about in this part of the book

The biggest difference between the two groups of people who made the change and followed the tips and advice written in the book are those people who have a very clear reason and are willing to do what is needed to deal with the situation. They have a very strong reason that they are willing to do a lot to change the point of life they are in.

There are two forces that can motivate a person to act. The first one is the avoidance of pain, and the second one is the attraction to pleasure. These two forces cause a person to make a change in his life. The great majority of people do their actions in life by avoiding pain. They stopped smoking, because the doctor told them that if they continued, they would die very quickly.

The same thing applies to being overweight. People get into a very difficult health condition before they are ready to make a change and, many times, they don't make a change until after a very traumatic event, such as a heart attack. They push themselves to the point where the suffering can no longer be tolerated, so there must be a significant change. Once they have experienced enough pain and fear, they will likely not return to the same place. On the other hand, those who simply decided that they only want to lose weight without a specific reason, have a much lower chance of success, because the person who has experienced the pain knows what to expect in the near future in the event he does not change his lifestyle now.

Does change equal suffering?

So, am I saying that the only way for you to make a significant change in your lifestyle is to go through a trauma or a crisis?

It is not possible to use those powers without knowing them. As soon as a person knows them and understands them in depth, he will discover forces he has not known until now, and these forces will help him and enable him to change the life of his children, himself, and his family.

In my opinion, this is the most important part of the book, and this is the reason I chose to put this information at the beginning. You need to open up and see what motivates you to action. If you do, your life will no longer look the same. So, I invite you to be part of this chapter. Please give it all the attention you need and use the tasks offered during the book.

What is your "why"?

The "why" is the biggest turning point a person can make for himself on almost any subject. A person who does not have a strong enough "why" will not be able to touch the same forces that will drive him to action, and he will simply remain in his comfort zone. The problem is that you should not expect things to change when you are in the center of your comfort zone, and you are not ready to push yourself into new boundaries. Once a person is willing to try new things and do tasks he has not done to date, he creates a new movement in his life. The same movement that did not exist until now causes the expansion of your comfort zone. I do not ask you to jump straight into the deep water. There is no need to turn your life into something completely different from what you are used to. Here is the power of gradualism. This gradualness will allow you to stretch your comfort zone a bit more without leaving it altogether. The power of "why" can give a person the power to move and create different results and expand their comfort zone.

How do you discover the "why"?

Your "why" usually sits very close to your heart. Once you find your "why," you will feel it in your body, your pulse will rise, and your body sensations will change. It may be a feeling similar to excitement or even the feeling that you are boarding a roller coaster. Usually, you don't get to that stage right from the beginning, because your brain is involved and giving its answers. But, like I said, it will be found very close to your heart, and it cannot be found the moment you look for the answers in your head. But, the answers you get from your head in the beginning will help you to slowly get close to your heart and find your real "why."

How does it work?

You have to ask yourself the right questions and answer them honestly. Once you are honest with yourself, you can give answers from the bottom of your heart. The power of those answers can change your life. One of the best ways I can define them is to find the same reasons for self-questioning. Self-questioning allows you to discover what is hidden in the depths of your mind, and you can discover what your real desires are.

In the next part of the chapter, I will ask you a question and you will answer it. Take it slow and give yourself all the time necessary to answer the question. In the exercise book, I wrote a partial exercise to perform the full exercise, which includes repeating the question seven times. This is the recommended amount required to go deeper and reach the real "why" found in your heart.

The full exercise can be found in the workbook.

Download the attached workbook. The download link is at the beginning of the book.

Even if you just do that part of the book, from my point of view, I did the work.

This is one of the most significant and important parts of the book. So let's get started!

What is the main reason you decided to read this book?

_____

_____

_____

_____

_____

_____

_____

Now that you have put your answer on the page, I want you to read it again and see what it makes you feel when you think about "why" that theme is so important to you and why you chose this reason. The goal is to get a little deeper into things and not talk straight from the head, and I want you to write here why you chose this topic.

_____

_____

_____

_____

_____

_____

_____

The deeper the question becomes, the more honest your answer will be. What usually happens is that the first questions we answer come from the head. As we mentioned earlier, the deeper you go, the more the answer will come, not from your head, but from your heart. I want us to go down another step. If you notice, they may bring you feelings that did not exist before you started the exercise. Now, I want you to write "why" you answered what you answered and whether this is the real reason for that answer. Are you avoiding something, or do you fear something that makes you want the same goal? Whatever the root of that choice is, what is the motive?

_____

_____

_____

_____

_____

_____

_____

In order to complete this exercise, you will need to continue it in the workbook.

Now, I want to ask you how you think your life will be if you can make a change about the same thing you chose for your "why." How will your life be after you go with your will and your heart? What will be different in your life? These questions will help you get to know the things that motivate you with pleasure.

_____

_____

_____

_____

_____

_____

_____

And, on the other hand, what will your life look like if you do not make the change you wish for? What happens if you continue to do the same things you did today? What happens if you stay in the same place that you and your family are in at this moment? What are the consequences of staying in the same place and not making a change in your life and that of your family? What could happen? What can you lose? This question will help you get to know the things that motivate you.

_____

_____

_____

_____

_____

_____

_____

After you have properly defined your "why," you may be aware of feelings you have not had until now. These same sensations will help you stick to your goal and do what is necessary to make that change in your family's life. This exercise is, in my opinion, a *must* before any change you want to make in life, because it helps you to know yourself better and helps you discover the real reasons that make you want to change. The more you get into the depth of your *why*, the more powerful this exercise and its impact on your life will be. This is not an exercise that has to be completed by a certain time. It can take days or weeks and many times the answers change. The exercise can be repeated over and over again to help you get closer to your answer.

If you have printed the attached booklet as recommended, you would put it nearby and periodically look in the book to see if you need to make changes or if you still identify with everything you have written.

I wish you great success. I truly believe that you can create a significant change in the life of you, your children, and your family.

The next chapter is, in my opinion, one of the most fascinating subjects. We will talk about the hidden mind. What is hidden behind the needs of the mind? We will understand better the language that the mind speaks, and we will know how to work with it in cooperation.

Chapter 2:
Body
and
mind

Where does it all begin?

Why are people overweight? The most common answer we hear is: a lot of food and a bit of activity. Is this the real problem of obesity or is it just the symptoms?

There is no doubt that overeating and inactivity lead to obesity. It cannot be disputed, but if it is true, a change in nutrition and physical activity would suffice and create the change that would last over time.

Nutrition combined with exercise is not enough to make a profound change and, in most cases, after a year, most people give up and return to their old habits and their initial weight. In order to create a change to the depth first, one must understand where the problem originates or what the emotional deficit is. Once the underlying cause is treated, it is possible to start using different ways to support the process and to do it correctly and in a balanced way, such as exercise and nutrition. For example, if you have weeds that fill the whole garden and you want them to disappear completely, because they just bother you, then grow flowers.

So, if your goal is to get rid of those weeds, will it be enough just to cut them down to get rid of them altogether?

A few weeks after you cut those weeds, they will grow again and take over the garden again. If you really want to get rid of those weeds, what you have to do is uproot them from the soil.

Once you have uprooted them, they will not grow again. Only then will you have the opportunity to create something new in the land that was occupied by the same weeds that disturbed you ... and all that remains to do is plant the right seeds and give them sun and water to grow abundantly.

Symptoms of eating disorders

- High body weight—although it seems that you eat little in public, you eat secretly
- Body weight changes frequently
- Lack of social and physical activity
- Physical problems such as shortness of breath, joint pain, excessive sweating, high blood pressure, etc.
- Hiding food for later consumption
- Eating large amounts of food without complaining of hunger or signs of hunger is the same condition usually accompanied by a lack of self-control in quantities
- Eating rate is generally higher
- Feelings of depression and guilt after uncontrolled eating

If you notice an eating disorder or behavioral change, first of all, call the child and ask what she's going through. There's probably a reason she behaves the way she does. Ask what bothers her and what she wants. Show her that you are interested in her and really want to understand her.

It is important to show interest all the time and not just when the child changes her behavior or her mood. Being interested in your child is something that needs to be daily and permanent. Building and developing such communication skills can take time and you need to be patient. If this is something that doesn't happen all the time, it is reasonable to assume that the child built a protective layer around herself. In order to reach it, you will need to peel off the shells slowly. Do not expect the child to open after the first shell. The child will probably not reveal all her cards. Be loving and attentive to the child's needs, give her the time she needs to open up, and be there for her.

There is no need to go through all of this alone. Consultation with a psychologist or childcare therapist can help guide and advise you about the situation the child is in. Do not get discouraged, and call for help if necessary.

Overeating disorder or compulsive eating

Compulsive eating is a disorder characterized by unbridled eating, and it's not because the food is particularly tasty. Eating is manifested in binge eating attacks that usually don't stop until the patient feels that he is unable to bring more food into the body. This can lead to a situation in which the person will experience severe body sensations and even a feeling of suffocation. People who suffer from compulsive eating disorder will not lead to emptying. This means that they will not vomit, as is common in patients with anorexia and bulimia.

The compulsive eaters use food as a way to cope with stress, emotional conflicts, and daily problems. Compulsive eating usually begins in early childhood when patterns of eating are shaped. Most people who become compulsive eaters are people who have never learned proper ways of dealing with stressful situations and, instead, use food as a way of coping. The more they gain weight, the more they try to diet, and the diet usually leads to the next binge, which can be accompanied by feelings of helplessness, guilt, shame, and failure.

What is emotional eating?

Older children and almost everyone else uses food to fill emotional deprivation. Eating can help dull and blur feelings and emotional states that are difficult for the child or adult to deal with, such as loneliness, anxiety, fear, stress, etc. For many people, eating in these situations serves as a defense mechanism that allows them to cope with those situations. When the adult or child feels that his feelings are moving toward the feelings that are less pleasant to experience, he will use food to feel better with himself or with the situation he encounters.

These feelings are short-lived and are not "real." These feelings that arise during eating "help to cope" for a short time with the same situation by raising the person's mood and distracting him from thinking about the things that bothered him or worried him. The thing is that after that person returns to the state he felt before eating, an act of emotional eating can soon become an addictive habit both in children and in adults who will repeat the same action again and again for the purpose of relaxation, compensation, etc.

This emotional eating is usually accompanied by a large consumption of sugars and other carbohydrates, which will eventually lead to obesity and all the symptoms that accompany it. The problem with those foods whose constant consumption causes full feelings of satisfaction is the constant exposure of the body to the hormones secreted during the consumption of those foods. This situation can be likened to a snowball that is located on a snowy slope.

The same situation of increased consumption of these foods will lead the person to consume more from time to time. In order to reach the same sense of satisfaction experienced in the beginning, the quantity will have to increase both in terms of times and in terms of quantities. The satisfaction will decrease, and the need to eat more and more will grow. Just as people addicted to alcohol and drugs raise the bar of their consumption each time to feel the same satisfaction, the same increase happens with emotional eating.

There is no such thing as a specific amount of attention or time that will help a child to overcome their emotional eating. Every child is different, and every child has to go through the process until he feels at peace with himself. As long as that circle does not close and the child does not feel at peace with the same subject, he should receive the necessary attention on that subject. Any emotion can be present, not just fear. Of course, not everything depends on the parent. It also depends on the child's ability to share these issues.

Recognize children's feelings and avoid feeling suppression

So, what are the consequences of suppressing feelings?

It is important to understand that the pain does not really disappear; it is only repressed from the awareness. Emotional suppression is not a complete action. It means that a person has repressed a subject from his life; it does not mean that it doesn't exist. He may consciously no longer remember that event and the emotions associated with it but, subconsciously, the event still exists, and it can lead to a constant state of tension, anxiety, and a sense of stress that causes mental fatigue.

Repression may be expressed in nightmares and sleep disorders because, during sleep, a person is fully connected to his subconscious. In addition, in many cases, the reason the repression occurs is because the person feels helpless and is unable to cope with reality or the situation. Over time, the same situation can lead to depression. Emotional suppression can lead to *hypersensitivity* once an emotion is suppressed and not dealt with. As a result, the next time the child encounters a similar situation, the reaction will be much stronger.

Emotional suppression and emotional numbness

When a child does not express their negative feelings, it can lead to suppressed sensations. This means that once the child does not express these feelings, the lack of expression of that emotion will cause the child not to express other emotions as well. The reason is that all emotions go through the same way. The moment a person blocks the negative emotions, the positive feelings are blocked and not experienced. It's like taking a pipe and just reducing the size of the opening on one side. Less dirt may enter but, on the other hand, less water will flow. It is therefore very important to let the child express all the emotions that arise in him because everything has a place. Anger, anxiety, happiness, and all the other emotions have a place for expression, and it is very desirable that everyone gets to express them.

Suppression of feelings and obesity

There are those who argue that suppression of emotions also creates an increased physiological tendency to store fat because that person is in a state of chronic stress. This causes an increase in cortisol hormones in the blood, which have a direct relationship to obesity. The issue of suppressing feelings is also true for children who have higher self-confidence and even more if their self-confidence is low. If the child is offended or harmed by a teacher, friend, or even a parent, it is important to give him room to express the feelings he has.

Become interested

The secret is simply to be interested in what caused him to feel the same feeling, whether it is the only thing he feels, or if there are any other things he feels. Ask the child what he expected to be different and why he was disappointed.

As you get more interested over time, the child will share with you more easily and by himself without you having to squeeze out every ounce of information.

Food as a resource

As we understand, eating has a great influence on our feelings, and a person can feel that eating serves as an emotional compensation, it is a warm and comforting member. Eating has a very large place in the life of that person. This means that the same food serves as a resource for that person. A resource can be a particular action or something in the life of the person who helps and promotes it. A resource for a particular person could be dancing, so, dancing could help that person.

In difficult moments, or in any situation where they have the need to cling to something, they will just go dancing. The resource has the power to make a person continue to progress despite the difficult things he is going through. A resource can serve as a kind of protective blanket that protects them.

Some people have turned to food as a resource. As you can imagine, this is not the ideal resource, because it has many health and mental implications. If a parent notices that their child turns to food as a resource every time, it is their role to help the child find new resources that will replace the resource that does not serve the child best, in this case, eating.

Replacing resources is very common in detoxification from various addictions like cigarettes, alcohol, and drugs. These addictions serve the person as a resource that enables them to ease the disengagement, etc. Although the resource may be similar (for example, smoking) the need it provides for one person is different from the need of another person. Although the action is the same, for one person smoking can be a quality time when they can disconnect from all the noise around them, and, for someone else, smoking may give a person a sense of popularity and a feeling of relevance.

Resource replacement

First of all, it is important to note that, in the process of replacing the resource, it is important to choose a resource that cannot cause damage and has positive advantages, because we do not intend to replace the resource again. For everyone to have their own personal resources, what needs to be done is to do a test with the child and see what things he likes to do. For example, does he like to paint, or sing, or dance? Does he like to ride a bike? There can be many options.

The goal is to find a resource that is subject to the eating resource, that is, if eating serves as a resource of relaxation and traveling by bicycle is also relaxing, this is an overlapping resource, and its use will be very helpful. In this case, the alternative resource is also easy to implement and accessible and, on the other hand, it has no harmful consequences.

Finding these overlapping resources can sometimes take time, and the best way to find those resources is to talk. Talk with the child and ask him what he likes and why he likes to do the activities. Once you have found the resource, and you think that resource can be an alternative for the child, encourage the child to use that resource more often.

So, if the child's resource is dancing, put strong music on, start dancing, and invite him to join you. The more he gets used to doing it, the more it will become a more accessible and achievable resource for him, rather than something that requires thought and effort. The more the child is exposed to another beneficial alternative, the less food they will need. If you see that the child is turning to food as a resource, it is possible to offer the same activities that can serve the child as a resource. It is true that the brain will create new connections in the brain and will understand that it has another way of dealing with the same situation and that food is not the only option.

Different types of emotional eating

Attract attention with eating disorders

Another reason for an emotional state that can benefit from eating is that the child feels that he is "transparent" or "no one sees him." If the child feels a lack of response and attention, it can create a feeling of emptiness in the child that he translates into a feeling of hunger. And what he does is fill that emptiness with food to feel full. The same obesity created by eating and changing eating is a mechanism that works in the subconscious mind of the child to "take a place" and be seen!

The same mechanism works for the other side in anorexia and bulimia. It is possible that the parent did not change anything in the way they behaved or in the amount of time they invested in their child. The only thing relevant in this case is how the child feels. This phenomenon can sometimes occur when a new child is born into the family or some other event happens. These events can be significant for the child. The child is afraid that his place is caught, and the purpose of the child is to be seen. The same eating disorder is usually accompanied by a change in behavior and an attempt to attract more attention than usual.

Eating in secret

Many of the occult eating cases may only be a boundary check, or an act of mischief, not something that needs to be addressed. Eating in secret is relevant in children and adults. Sometimes, eating in secret only means that you do not want to share your candy, and you eat it alone without sharing it with the rest of the people or the family around. Eating in secret can also arise simply because there is no desire to hear comments from family or friends. ("What an amazing amount of weight you've lost. Why do you need it now?)

So, when should a red light turn on?

When you notice that eating in secret becomes a habit that repeats itself time after time or that eating in secret becomes the preferred way of eating meals during the day, this is the moment when the red light is supposed to turn on. The more alert the parent is to the child, the more they will be able to observe and avoid the eating disorder in advance. The fact is that it is not always possible to observe the same state of secret eating, because this phenomenon is often characterized by compulsive eating of small portions that do not appear to be serious.

But, what I suspect is that it goes on all day long and eventually the consumption of calories is higher than what is needed for the body, which ultimately leads to a positive calorie balance that causes obesity. Usually, those foods are not nutritious and do not require any kind of preparation. Most often, they are snacks or things that are already ready and packed so that they can be eaten in secret, without anyone noticing. It must be remembered that eating in secret is not as easy for a child as for an adult. A lot of energy is invested into hiding the food, so that the parents do not notice what he eats or when he eats. He has to remove the evidence and eat fast, and he may even have to invent stories and start to lie.

Significant events in life and emotional eating
Significant life events that cause stress can affect the child's or the adult's mental state.

For example, a war or the death of a close person or a pet can be experienced as traumatic. It does not necessarily have to be traumatic, but an extreme change can lead to eating disorders if they are not prepared for the change. It may be a transition that can be considered a significant and even traumatic event for some children, like changing locations, changing schools, and leaving friends. This sharp transition can lead to a situation where he feels unrepentant and has no ability to control what is happening in his life. If the parent does not notice it at the time, it can lead to emotional eating. This emotional eating will help the child cope in such a way that it will help him deal with what he is feeling, and the food can now serve him as a new member (since he is far from his friends). A life event that is considered significant for one child may be considered unbearable for another child.

Pre-preparation and elimination of uncertainty
One of the ways to deal with significant events in life, for example, by moving to an apartment, is to prepare in advance. You can go to the area where you intend to move. You can go with the children to one of the gardens in the area and even take a small trip to the schools in the area.

One of the main things that make the situation so traumatic is the uncertainty associated with the transition. Once the child has seen the area, has seen the neighborhood parks and schools, and he has seen possible new friends, it can significantly help make the move to a new area easier. The very act of talking about the subject, listening to the child's fears, and having a conversation with the child about these issues will help him cope and get ready for the change. The lack of reference to these feelings or their suppression can lead to many consequences, one of which is emotional eating.

What can prevent emotional eating?

Communicate with the child

Communication is the most basic thing for a healthy relationship between parents and children. If communication has failed, it is not good, and it can harm the trust between the child and the parents. This is accompanied by a lack of openness. The whole situation creates a situation that makes it very difficult for parents to find out where the child's emotional deprivation is, what state he is in, and what he wants.

As the gap between the parent and the child grows and the subject is not dealt with, it will cause the child to gather more and more within himself and build more defenses. When there is good communication between parents and children, trust and closeness are strengthened. This creates a healthy communication that enables the child to express himself and ask for the things he wants. For the communication to be of good quality, it is always important to be careful to talk to the child at eye level.

Once the child feels that it is okay to say what he feels or wants, he will have more confidence to talk and share more about himself.

Improving the skill of conversation between parent and child

- *Ask* - ask your child about his day more often and really listen.
- *Ask open-ended questions* - try to ask more open questions, which will make it possible to develop a conversation with your child and make it difficult for them to answer yes or no. For example, asking the question "how was school today?" is not enough because her answer could just be "good," "okay," or "boring." Answers that amount to one or two words are not enough. Ask questions that invite you into the conversation. Ask more profound questions to help you understand what is going on.
- *Ask them about their feelings* - talk to them about their difficulties and the things they enjoy doing. Ask about the people they love and how those people make them feel. Ask them about the things they told you a day or two ago, and it will show them that you really listen to them and think about what they told you. The following is an example of some open questions whose answer will require more than one word.

For example, instead of asking how he was at school, you can ask if he played with Jim, or if they have gotten back together after their fight yesterday, how it felt seeing him again, etc. Beyond the fact that these questions allow for a more profound answer, these questions allow the child to share with the parent what he feels and thinks, and that helps him develop more conversationally. It is very important to maintain consistency. Consistency creates trust between parent and child. It shows the child that the parent is there for him and always will be, and that the parent is really interested in him and how he feels. Over time, you will be surprised how this little change will build trust and change your relationship.

Love

Love is the most basic element.
In order for the child to grow and develop in a healthy way, he needs to receive love. The child should feel loved. A sense of love should be familiar to him, and it is essential for the healthy development of a child. A child who feels loved builds a higher self-confidence and a stronger character, and it allows him to grow up with the feeling that he is equal. Bringing love to a child will make the child grow up feeling that his parents will always be there for him when he needs them. The love received will make him a better person, and he will not be afraid to ask them what he needs. And, of course, once a child knows what love is and how love should be, he can know for himself how to express the feeling of love. Receiving love will teach him how to give love.

"All you need is love, all you need is love, love, love is all you need..."-The Beatles

---

70

A rejected child

One of the most difficult traumas a child can experience is rejection by his parents, especially by his mother. Not all parents know how to give love, and not all parents love their children equally. Some parents feel that their children are a burden in their lives. Of course, not everything is rosy all the time and all parents sometimes feel frustrated, distressed, tired, and exhausted. It is perfectly legitimate and logical. Raising children is not easy and requires great effort.

But the problem is that many times, because of all the attention that goes into raising children, many parents forget their own personal needs. A parent may feel that the child is a burden, and that may lead to resentment. It may even lead to the parents being repulsed by the children and, in extreme situations, it can lead to verbal and physical abuse. The issue is that those parents who experience this have difficulty providing themselves with what they need personally, while, at the same time, giving their children constant love and security. These parents tend to be disorganized, self-centered, impulsive, and hot-tempered.

Lack of love during childhood

Everyone now knows that if children do not get certain vitamins in their early years—like vitamins A, B, or D—they will have skeletal problems and other health problems until they die. So, there is a very controlled follow-up on what a child should have in his early years to grow healthy.

Lack of love will cause a disability, not physically but emotionally. The damage done to the child is sometimes irreversible and cannot be dealt with or solved completely. But, in many cases, it is possible to treat the adult. The thing is that this person will have to make great efforts to work on the deprivation created during his life and, of course, it will leave many scars.

Biologically, the brain patterns of children who have been neglected or abused or have not received enough love differ from those of children who have received love. For example, neglected babies have higher levels of cortisol, a hormone that affects metabolism in the body, which is excreted in increased stress, and lower levels of oxytocin (a stress reliever) associated with the formation of a "social connection." The high levels of cortisol cause children to feel anxious about people. Consequently, they grow up feeling afraid they will get hurt by people and, therefore, do not rush to trust them. They always feel that something is wrong with them.

Today, more and more hospitals are hosting entire teams of volunteers whose job is to give love to those abandoned babies in hospitals. Studies show that children who are not exposed to love at the beginning of their lives are much more exposed to mental problems and adjustment to adoptive families.

In addition to this, newborns who were abandoned in the hospital who did not receive warmth and love were sick more often and even died as a result of this deficiency. We can hear of cases of death in the wake of grief, although this is not the same case, but one can see the resemblance between these cases. These cases show you what the power of love is and how it can affect your children. So, what are you waiting for? Give a warm hug to your kids and tell them how much you love them!

- Be sure to tell them how much you love them
- Show them that you love them unconditionally
- Show them that you love them even when they "fail" or make mistakes in their actions
- Be sure to tell them often, "You're special to me. I will always love you, no matter what!"
- Teach them respect for all the things that are good, and compliment them as often as possible.

The importance of *seeing* your children

What do I mean by saying "see" your children?
The meaning of this phrase is not necessarily to see your children physically. But the intention is that he or she has a place, that you pay attention to her and what she has to say, and that she can decide and express her opinions. Talk to her at eye level. Of course, every age has their understanding ability. The feeling that you see her for the child she is is very important. When a child feels that you "see" them and you relate to them and their desires, their self-confidence will be higher, and they will feel that they are valued and they have a place and importance. She will feel more confident in herself, and it will affect her in many ways. A child who feels that their parents actually "see" them is much less likely to produce dramas for attention.

73

Avoid ignoring and silencing

This situation is very common when the parent is busy. The child turns to the parent and the parent waves the child away because they are in the middle of something important or busy with a conversation. The flapping can hurt a child very much, because a child does not really understand why they waved him away. He cannot make the calculation that his parent is busy, that he cannot express what he wants at that moment, and that the parent ignores him.

The inability to express oneself can reduce the child's self-confidence or harm the parent-child trust. Of course, this doesn't happen after one incident but, if the child feels that he is rejected every time, it will create a stronger sense of rejection. His self-confidence will decline, and he will feel that he is not seen.

So, how do you act in such a situation without harming your child?

1. Stop the conversation for a second, and tell the other side to wait a few seconds.
2. Drop to the height of your child's eyes and explain to the child in a calm and listening way that you really want to hear but you are in the middle of an important conversation and that once you are done, you will listen to her or play with her or anything else that the child asked for. In most cases, you stopped what you were doing, gave your attention, and your heart did the rest. And the child will not feel ignored or unwanted.
3. Go back and continue to conduct the conversation as usual.
4. End the call.

5. Return to the child.

Beyond the fact that you have earned your child's respect and that the child understands that you see her, I am sure that the person on the other side of the line will greatly appreciate the way you responded to that situation in a responsible and tolerant manner, which ultimately earned you two birds with one stone.

Their opinion is important

Everyone likes to give their opinion, and children also want to give their opinion. An expression of opinion leads to a sense of belonging. So, ask their opinion on many issues and ask what they think about it. At first, the child will not participate. And that makes sense, especially if it's something that has not happened until now. But this simple action can build an improved and upgraded relationship that includes love, caring, acceptance, and listening.

When you are with them, *be* with them

There are parents who are with their children all day, and some parents arrive home late after a long day's work.

Which parent is considered better?

Is it the parent who has been with their children all day?

The amount of hours the child spends with the parent is of no importance. The question is *how* the parent spends their time with the child. One parent may only spend an hour with his child, but he gives his full attention to the child, playing with him and listening to him. It is only him and the child. On the other hand, a parent who spends many hours at home can find himself playing with Sonny to relax, and Sonny benefits greatly from this one-on-one association.

The amount of time doesn't matter. What really matters is *how* the parent spends the time with his children. It doesn't matter if you have one hour or five hours; it is the way you spend that time with your child. So, do not mess with anything other than them—no phone, no TV, no Facebook. Give them 100 percent of your attention.

If you don't do it and you don't really give them the full attention they deserve, you will get up one day and realize that you missed so many years when you were not really present for them. They needed you more than anything, and you missed so many beautiful moments for things that will feel meaningless to you in the future. In addition to all this, imagine how insulting and offensive it is to talk to someone when the person you're talking to looks at TV with one eye and browses Facebook with the other eye while you're trying to talk to them. It would probably bother you very much, and it would feel you were being disrespected and not being listened to. This is what the child feels when he thinks that he isn't being given your full attention. If you think the kids don't notice, I have news for you. They pay attention to every step you take, and they will know that you are not completely with them.

Chapter 3:
Habits
and
environment

The early years

The first six years of the child's life are critical to shaping his personality. In his early years, the child learns about himself and what he is capable of. He knows his abilities during these years, and he develops his own beliefs. He begins to see himself in a certain way, wonders if is he is loved, if he is seen, etc.

After 6 years of age, the child begins to compare himself to his environment. This stage happens upon entering school. A child whose base is not stable enough and self-confidence is low will have a harder time coping with things he will encounter during his life. However, a child who has the tools to deal with the things life brings to him will deal better.

A child who does not have the necessary tools to cope with the real world will begin to encounter situations in the school that will be very difficult to cope with and, over the years, the situation will get worse if he is not treated. The child will grow up with a sense of incompetence, and he will have a low self-image and low body image. All these situations can lead to overweight and obesity.

The parent has the ability to construct and change the way the child sees himself with the right intention of seeing the whole picture and imparting healthy habits to the child. The parent is the child's guide, and the parent can change the child's life and shape the personality in the future. Even if the child has passed the age of 6, it does not mean that this situation is over; it will just be a bit more challenging. The parent has the ability to build a happy and healthy child who knows how to deal with life and is prepare for real life. The thing is that this topic has so many parameters and so many opinions that it can be very confusing and make it difficult for the parent to make the right choice. In this chapter, I have focused on the main themes of designing a good environment and healthy habits for your child to fulfill his full potential.

The power of a personal example

The parent has a significant role in shaping the child emotionally and physically. In addition, a parent is a child's role model. Do not expect your children to do things that you do not do on your own.

A personal example is worth much more than a thousand words. A personal example is a key tool in shaping the personality of the child, and a lot of the personality of the child is built from observing the actions of the parent. It is important to remember that we are all human beings and sometimes we are wrong, but the most important thing is to really give our best and improve every day knowing that your child is watching.

The child learns from the actions of the parent. If a child grows up in a violent environment, for example, it does not necessarily mean that violence was directed at the child herself. It is enough that she observes the behavior she sees around herself. This is what she will see fit to do, and she will become a child who acts violently and aggressively to those around her and, in many cases, she will become a violent adult. This whole situation happens as the child imitates her immediate environment.

The same thing is true about sports and nutrition. A child who grows up in the environment of a family of athletes—who enjoy training and living a healthy life where sports is a hobby that takes a significant part of the way the family spends their time—is likely to grow up as a child who likes to do sports and will always want to take part in the activity and even initiate it herself. The parent must aspire to behave in their own life as they would like their children to behave, to the smallest details.

The child as a mirror

Reflection can come in several forms of mirroring an emotional state and reflecting a behavioral state. As soon as you recognize that something is wrong or you dislike the child's behavior, you should first check to see if it is reflected from you. Are you bothered lately by work and getting more nervous and perhaps not giving the child enough attention? Are you becoming impatient and just want it quiet when you get home? These are questions that can help you examine the situation.

For example, if the father is very troubled by a promotion he did not receive, he goes home with the same bad feeling. For a few days, he may have thought that he would get the raise he wanted, and he planned how it would help him close the mortgage. The child can reflect the same concern and feelings that the father felt, and the child will be less focused on his studies and may be restless or even dreamy. The child identifies with the same feelings that the father feels.

Another example is the father's annoyance. "He has a short fuse." He may never have raised his voice at his children or his wife, but the child can still distinguish the same behavior in those around him, whether it is on the road, in the grocery store, or in other different situations. The child can reflect this behavior because he thinks it is the right behavior—he should behave this way because that is what he learned from his father.

Once you notice something like this, first look at yourself to see whether it is a result from your action or behavior. Could your child have learned it from you without you noticing?

It's important to remember
Every day is a new day, so if you lose it one day, it's okay. Always remember that Rome was not built in a day. It takes time to build new habits. Be patient and you will enjoy the positive consequences of those new habits you adopted for yourself and your family.

The parent is allowed to make a mistake
It is very important to give up the ego in these things if you have come to a situation where you feel that you have raised your voice too much or ignored your child's feelings. It is very important that you admit your mistake to yourself too, but it is especially important that you share it with your child. Tell her that you regret that you have hurt her and you will work on yourself so that situation will not happen again.

"Children have never been attentive to their parents, but they have never stopped imitating them, they must, they have no other models." – James Baldwin

Parent as leader

In addition to the fact that a parent should be a personal example for a child in the process of transitioning to a healthy diet and a healthy lifestyle, they should harness the whole family to the same process and, of course, continue to be a personal example and lead the same movement. In the event that the parent does not take control of the family's change, there will be a split in the home—those who have passed through to a healthy lifestyle and those who have not.

For example, if the family's aim is to help one of the family members to lose weight, they should not put the one child on a diet and tell them what they are allowed and what they are not allowed to eat while the rest of the people at home eat what they like, because they are not overweight. This situation can cause a lot of problems for the child. First, it will make the child feel irrelevant and discriminated against. A child cannot understand it as you understand it. They do not see it as something in their favor.

In such a situation, the child feels that he has been wronged, and that makes him feel that he is unusual and different from everyone, and they treat him differently because of this. Believe me, he feels very different from everyone else. The child's environment reminds him of that. Even then, there is no need to differentiate him at home. It is very important that the whole house do this process together. The parents are the ones at the head of this task. The parents should not set a diet for just one child, as this will make your child hate diets and proper nutrition for their entire life, because it makes them feel different and unusual.

Self-Confidence

Self-esteem is a term in psychology that describes the emotional assessment of the value of the human being. This means how a person sees himself and the way he comes to attribute to himself. Self-esteem is manifested in a number of mental levels:

- In perception (e.g., "I am talented" or "I am valuable")
- Feelings (such as despair, pride, shame)
- Behavior

Self-esteem is the negative or positive assessment of the self, in the sense of the characteristics of feelings that one feels toward oneself. The experiences that a person experiences during their lives are central to the development of self-esteem and self-confidence. The same negative or positive life experience creates the way that person comes to look at life and itself.

You can look at past experiences as glasses that let you reflect on childhood as the internal and external world you see. Now the question is which glasses will you bring your kids?

One way would be to develop healthy feelings of self-worth, and the opposite way is developing negative feelings about self-worth. In early childhood, parents are the most important influence on a child's self-esteem, and the parent is the strongest source of positive or negative experiences that the child will experience during his early life.

Self-confidence is a very important and the basic component of a happy life, and there are many components that cause feelings of security and belonging. A person can be very talented and have amazing character traits but, if his confidence is very low, it can hurt him despite all the good qualities that are in him including his skills. Low self-confidence can make it difficult on many issues in life.

Negative body image and self-love

So, what is a body image? A body image is the way a person perceives the appearance of his body and how others perceive his body. So, if a person sees himself as ugly, he thinks that the whole world sees him in the same way that he sees himself, even though people can see him as handsome and attractive.

Body image is directly related to your general self-image and self-confidence and actually begins to build up in early childhood. However, self-image can change during your life, for better or for worse. The older a person gets, the more he is affected by what is happening around him, from television publications and characters, and the ideal look is built in his head.

The more the child is affected by the environment, the better/worse his/her body image will be. Although the body image begins to show its signs in the early years of childhood, it can be seen more clearly when the child reaches the 6-7 age zone. This is the same period when the child begins to compare himself to others at the beginning of school. Sex has an important self-image, and studies conducted on this subject show that women tend to have a lower body image than men do.

"I'm not what I think I am. I'm not what he thinks I am. I'm what I think he thinks I am."-
Unknown

Negative body image usually does not disappear just like that, and it accompanies the person throughout his life. In many cases, the low body image gets stronger over the years, and that can lead to mental problems and various difficulties such as depression, self-hatred, eating disorders, anxieties, neglect of appearance, avoiding social situations, etc. The parent has a great influence on the child's self-image and takes a significant part in this matter.

Personal example: What is a healthy and positive body image?

Imagine a mother who spends all day focused on her weight. She counts calories and weighs herself every day. And, every day she is afraid of becoming obese. She raises the same themes again and again in the children's surroundings, not necessarily telling them about how she feels about her body, but it's enough that they hear her saying such and such statements about her body, and that she is not pleased with it. These statements can manifest themselves in different forms like: I do not like my legs, I do not like my stomach, etc.

A child learns from a situation where the parent does not love his own body. A personal example of a self-image is a very important part, and it can have a great influence on how the child's body image will be constructed.

"If you really love your children, and they are important to you, and you just want them to feel good, be themselves, and love their bodies, then start by loving yourself!" –Bar Aizik

---

How to help your child build a positive self-image
Compliments - the more the parent does it, the more the child will see himself in the same way. It is important to remember that it is never too late to make a significant change in the way your children see themselves or you see yourself. It is best to start at an early age but, even at a later age, it is entirely possible.

Do you see your child?
A child sees his image according to the way he is reflected in his parents' eyes. If you see your child as a successful person, it is more likely that this will also be her experience. What you think about your child is what she will be.

If a parent feels confident about certain issues in the child, the child will probably feel it. In this way, the child will also feel secure about these situations or issues. On the other hand, a parent who feels uncomfortable about situations in which the children are less "good" or "hard-pressed," the child will feel the same and act with uncertainty.

The way the parent sees the child has a great influence on the child's feelings for several reasons

- One of the reasons is the parent's response. A parent who is stressed or afraid will act and perform actions to protect his son, so that he will not get hurt. This overprotection can create in the child a sense of inability to do things on his own.
- Another reason is that the child can pay attention to the feelings of the parent even without the parent saying a word or doing a certain action. The child can feel the insecurity of the parent. The child's intuition is well developed, and he will notice the emotional state found in the parent. This can lead to the child acting insecure and fearful, because that is what he experiences from the parent.

For example, if a parent sees the child as having a problem with socializing, as soon as the child is in a situation where he or she can have contact, the parent may feel a certain fear, because they don't want their child to be hurt or disappointed. But, what actually happens is that the child will notice that the parent is anxious or stressed, and that can lead to the child feeling insecure when he has the opportunity to make new connections.

As a result, if the same situation repeats itself again and again, that experience will grow and intensify, which can lead to the difficulty of creating social connections in the future. As you see the child as a child with a problem, the same problem will only continue to grow. This does not mean that one must ignore the difficulty, but it is not necessary to turn the difficulty that the child has into something that is part of him. The role of the parent is to help the child overcome the situation and give him the tools to deal with the difficulty and show him how good and amazing he is just as he is (without changing anything).

So, what do you do when your feelings are taking over?

First stage — observation
First of all, start by paying attention to what you are going through. What feelings are rising?

What happens to your body once your child is in the same situation that triggers you emotionally? From the moment you notice the physical and emotional state you are in, you have already done eighty percent of the work. The very fact that you notice what feelings arise in parallel to that situation, they cease to be in control of that situation and control is restored to you. From that moment, you can tell yourself that these are just feelings and that they no longer manage you.

Second stage — change the focus
Once you have identified that feeling, focus your attention on the good things you see in your child. What are all the

things she's good at? What makes her special? What features do you really like? This can help make a difference in the way you look at your child. That means, if you've been wearing black glasses for a particular situation, as soon as you adopt other feelings—the same good things you see in your child—it helps you change your glasses to pink glasses. The situation is the same situation but the way you will experience it will be different once you put on the pink glasses.

After being careful to give attention to the feelings that are going through you in those situations, change them to positive feelings. These positive feelings will become assimilated in the context of a situation that you previously saw as problematic.

It is a process that can take time, and it takes time to change the way you think and look at things, especially as those situations cause unpleasantness and interfere with your feelings. But that action can make a significant difference in your children's life, just because of the simple action you have done between yourselves.

Changing Thinking Patterns

As the years go by, the way the children see themselves is stabilized and shaped and a change will be more challenging. This means that if a child sees himself as not successful, or not talented, or not smart, the same feelings will only grow and expand over the years, and he will begin to believe those feelings. And, when he encounters situations that encourage what he previously thought of himself, it will build even more of his sense of a lack of success. Everyone has thoughts that make him afraid to make changes; everyone has some sort of image of himself.

Although many people tell him that thinking what he thinks of himself is not true, it is not enough. For years and years, people can find themselves trying to make a change in their way of thinking to create a new belief for themselves, because they know the power of those beliefs. A person has the ability to change their lives as a result of changing the way they see themselves or believe in themselves. As a result of this change, they can create a whole new life to act and do things they haven't done to this day. Many people turn to psychologists and holistic therapists and coaches to work on the same beliefs and patterns they want to change.

The parent can often be used as a "therapist." There is no need to study special training to be your child's counselor to help them change that limiting belief that is beginning to develop in them.

What should be done?
Listen - be attentive to their difficulties, their decisions, and the way they see life. One statement can change a person's life. A child with a low self-image tends to see things in his or her life in a negative and unsuccessful way, as if nothing succeeds. Help them overcome this way of thinking and give them the opportunity to see themselves in another light by strengthening the child's strengths and creating small successes on the same subject they sees themselves as unsuccessful. Remember that changing habits and

patterns of thinking takes time, so give it time until you see that same pattern of thinking has changed.

The steps to change a limiting belief

In order to make a change in their way of thinking, they need to go through stages. As soon as a child or adult passes through all these steps, they will have the opportunity to rid themselves of the old belief and adopt a new belief. This process could take months. Do not expect to solve it within an hour. In the end, it is a child and you want to help them as you move through it. The child does not have to feel that they are doing "work" here. Rather, all the steps that I am going to note should fit in as part of your day-to-day experiences with your child. The role of the parent in this process is to help the child to go through these steps on his own. The parent is only the navigator; the child is the pilot. The child must do the thinking on his own and produce the change himself.

1. Locate the current / limiting belief.
2. Start questioning this belief. ("Maybe what I thought up until now is not really as true as I thought.")
3. The abandonment of the old faith. ("I understand that this belief is really not true to me, and what I thought about that belief is not relevant today.")
4. To discern a new faith. ("What is the new faith that I want to adopt that can help me?")
5. To open up to the new faith. ("Perhaps what I thought was wrong or not related to me. It is true and connected to me, and there is a situation that I have not seen to this day.")
6. Add the new faith to my most basic belief system. ("I believe in my new faith and know that it is very true to me and that it is part of me, just as I know that if I touch a fire I will get burnt.")

Activate creativity and see how you can use the six steps to help your children change the faith they see in themselves, for example, they are not successful, they are not pretty, they are not smart, or anything else that hurts them. In addition, of course, it is always important to strengthen the issues in which the child is good, to encourage them often, and to create a sense of success in them, which will help them build their self-confidence.

Changing beliefs is a very big issue that requires time to learn. Be patient and deepen it as much as possible, and you can do wonders with it.

It's never too late

Even if your child has passed the age of six, these are the years that build most of your child's self-confidence. You can change this even at a later age. Give the child the feeling that all his successes depend on him and his abilities.

The story of Thomas Edison

"The greatest inventor of all time" attended school for only three months when he was seven, and he was expelled after the teachers decided there was no chance he could absorb the material. They thought he was too slow to study the material.

What caused the child who had difficulties in school to become the greatest inventor in history?

There are those who say that it was a combination of strong ambition and tremendous self-confidence.

But where did all his self-confidence come from, and where did it all begin?

After only three months, Thomas was thrown out of school and was given a letter for his mother. He was seven years old, and he didn't know how to read or write.

When Thomas's mother saw him at home so early in the day, she was surprised to see him with a letter in his hand. The same letter said, "Your child, Thomas Edison, is slow or even retarded, and he will not be able to attend school."

Thomas's mother choked with tears, took a deep breath, and started to read to Thomas what was written there. She looked into Thomas's confused eyes, smiled, and began to read again.

"Thomas Edison is a brilliant and smart child and the school cannot teach him because of his genius. Please teach him at home."

Thomas's mother understood, even then, how the information in the letter could be traumatic for her son. So, she took her son, built his self-confidence, so he would see himself as successful, and did whatever else it took to teach him the best she could, and she did it all at home.

Thanks to Thomas's mother, we won the greatest inventor in history.

Presumably, this is because of his mother, but one can thank the teacher who defined him as retarded. The parent has tremendous power in shaping the child's confidence and building his personality. Maybe your child will be the next Edison.

We will never know unless you help your child to reach his full potential.

Grow with a sense of competence

Competence is the ability to succeed. A child with high ability can gain success during his life more easily and, as a result, his self-image will rise. A child who has experienced failures during his life can attribute this to his lack of abilities, and his self-image will be damaged. People with low self-competence tend to believe that tasks are too complex for their abilities, they avoid coping with those difficulties, they are afraid of tasks that provide low motivation, they give up easily once obstacles arise, and they lose confidence in their abilities.

On the other hand, people with high self-competence tend to live with the sense that they believe in their ability to complete tasks, they look at difficulty as a challenge, they develop great interest in doing their tasks, they are motivated, they commit to completing the task, and they recover quickly after failure.

It is said that the most important source of competence development is the experience of completing tasks. When we succeed in carrying out a task, our self-efficacy rises and when we fail, it decreases. One way to build a sense of competence in children is to set small measurable goals or to define tasks that they can complete. The emphasis is on many small goals so that they can experience as many successes as possible.

Reinforcing self-confidence by setting goals
Setting goals is an amazing tool for creating self-confidence. One of the things that leads to the construction of self-confidence is repeated successes on

the same subject and vice versa—lack of successes on the same subject creates a sense of frustration and failure.

So, how can you create successes by setting goals?
The goal should be something that can really be achieved. Start small and help your child gain confidence, so that his self-confidence will gradually increase, and then you can raise the goal from time to time. Set goals that are appropriate for the child's age and abilities, because if you set an unattainable goal, it will have a negative effect.

As soon as you help the child achieve the goal, compliment him on his achievements, but mainly focus on the qualities that have contributed to his success and his actions to succeed. And, from time to time, you will be able to set up slightly larger goals for the child to help the child push himself more to succeed. This will help build the child's personality and self-confidence.

Self-confidence is like the roots of a tree. The more roots it has and the deeper they penetrate into the earth, the more stable the tree will be and the easier it will be for the tree's growth.

setting goals technique

One way to set goals is the S.M.A.R.T model. Many managers use this model to set goals. We will use this model to set goals for children.

Specific, detailed, and clear

If the goal is not clear enough, you will never know which direction you want to go. It's like telling a taxi driver that you want to go to New York City, but you don't give him the name of the street you want. The goal must be specific and clear to both the parent and the child. It is important for the child to understand exactly what the goal is. Once he knows clearly what the goal is, he will be able to adjust to it. Without clarity, it would be very difficult to reach the same goal.

Measurable

For a goal to be achieved effectively, it must be given a timeframe (or a starting line) and a finish line. If it is not clear where the beginning is and where the end will be, it will never be possible to know whether the mission was really carried out. So, once you decide to set an important goal, the child not only knows what the goal is, but she knows what she needs to do to keep on the right track. For example, we will take a child who begins to learn to ride a bicycle.

Purpose without measurement: Ride easily as many times as you want without falling.

Purpose with measurement: Ride continuously ten meters in a straight line.

*A*ttainable

It is very important that the goal be achievable, so you start with small goals. Big goals can stress the child and appear threatening. Therefore, it is very important to start small and, as time passes and self-confidence grows, it will be possible to raise the level in setting goals.

*R*ealistic

The goals must be challenging, and you will set goals with your child so that he is proud of them. Once the child has achieved the goal, he will experience a sense of ability and success. This means that if the child scores ten baskets in a row without a problem then this is not considered a challenge. However, if you set the goal to score fifteen baskets in a row, it is a little more challenging, it raises the level of difficulty, and it makes the goal realistic and challenging.

An unrealistic goal is to tell him to score 100 baskets in a row, which can lead to a sense of failure over and over, and that can lead to despair.

*T*ime Bound

The larger the goals, the more you will need to use that part of the formula. Timing is critical and important, and it helps motivation and action. If you set a goal but did not give it a final time limit, then, basically, it is possible to finish the same goal in two years, and it will be considered that the child has done the task. It is important to focus on larger goals that require more than a few minutes. It is important to note that the larger the goal, the better it is to break it down into smaller steps. You can see it like stairs and every step that goes up brings us closer to the goal. Breaking up the big goal into smaller targets is another way to measure progress toward the goal.

Every success is a family success

The whole family is part of the change. Look at yourself as a team, give your group a name, make costumes for everyone, and do a division of labor. It is much easier to achieve the goal as a group rather than as an individual. Teach your children the power of cooperation and support for each other within the family unit. A common mistake is to label one of the children as "fat."

The parents and the children must undergo the change together. Once they all work together, and they are ready for the same task, everyone will be successful, and not just for the purpose of one thing. It will create a sense of unity and family cohesion. A family that builds the family unity in a good way will create a sense of pride in the unit, just like in the army. The pride of the unit has a great influence on the soldier's performance within the military framework in terms of motivation to carry out the actions and concern for all the staff. It should be the same in a family, as there will be more pride in the family unit, the cooperation will be better, and the relationship will improve and be better for everyone.

Setting goals and objectives as a family
Setting goals is a powerful tool, and it should be understood how important this topic is in building the personality of a child.

Setting goals is a very good tool that gives a person the direction he wants to reach. A person without a clear goal will not get to where he wants to go. He may have moved in a certain direction, but it's not necessarily where he wants to go. Therefore, it is very important to create a clear goal before embarking on any action. A family that gets together for a certain purpose is much more powerful than just one person or only part of the house trying to achieve the same goal.

One of the things I enjoy most is seeing an entire family, all of whom are recruited for the same task. This cooperation creates better connections between the family members. It creates collaboration and improves communication. Setting goals as a family creates the feeling that everyone has their own importance and their share in the family, and it creates a sense of belonging that is something very basic and necessary for success.

Creating a family's goals

For the entire family to be recruited for the same task, it is very important that each and every member of the family understands the importance of the subject. The subject we are talking about in this book is creating a healthy and balanced family. So, the goal can be to become a healthy and balanced family within six months that eat healthy and exercise together several times a week. This will be the ultimate goal.

So, how do you recruit the whole family to this action?

1. Example - parents should be role models for children
2. Consent and cooperation between the parents
3. Commitment and consistency to the goal

If one parent aims to make the family healthy, and the other parent buys pizzas all the time, it means that there is a mismatch between the two sides. Therefore, it is very important that there be cooperation between the parents before they create a goal. The first step is always the parents. After they both agree and are willing to work together toward the same goal, they need to come to an understanding and ask all the family members why they all have to do this and why they all have to make the same change. We talked about "why" at the beginning of the book. If you did not do the exercise, it is recommended that you do it. It will help you greatly in determining your goal.

Once you have set your goal, you can start by setting small targets and first goals. The first goals are solely for the parents, and there is no need to involve the children. The goal is to set a personal example for the children. Children will see their parents doing something specific and making a change, and it will be easier for the kids to accept it. Asking a child to do a certain action, without the parent doing it too, can raise certain objections.

Setting a family goal step by step

The next exercise will help you implement your family goals and make them part of your family's lifestyle.

The full exercise can be found in the workbook. Set goals for the next three months.

Download the attached workbook. The download link is at the beginning of the book.

Goals for the next ninety days

What is the goal you want to achieve as a family over the next ninety days?

_____

_____

_____

_____

_____

_____

_____

Why is it so important to you?

_____

_____

_____

_____

_____

_____

The next step is the dismantling of a large goal into smaller targets that will help move towards the goal.

The first goal setting will be for the first week, and the actions are to be performed by the parents only.

During the coming week, choose a personal and a non-family goal. For example, start getting into shape, start eating more healthily, or any other habit you want to become a family thing.

My goal for next week is:

_____

_____

_____

_____

_____

_____

_____

Now, take that goal and break it down into smaller actions. What actions can you do during the week to start fulfilling the same goal that you have set for your entire family? For example, do a double walk this week for half an hour on Monday and Thursday. What is the goal for the coming week? What do you want to achieve? more exercise? eating healthier? etc.

What are the things that I am going to change in the next seven that I know I can handle? What are the things that, after I do them, I'll know I've succeeded?

_____

_____

_____

_____

_____

_____

After you've passed the first week, it's time to start expanding your goal and pick another small goal. Of course, you continue with the same actions you did the previous week.

My goal for Week # 2 is:

_____

_____

_____

_____

_____

_____

_____

_____

_____

What are the things that I am going to change in the next seven that I know I can handle? What are the things that, after I do them, I'll know I've succeeded?

_____

_____

_____

_____

_____

_____

After two weeks, you've already started moving toward your goals, and you're on a mission. It's time to share with your children the change you've begun to make in your personal life. Share with them not only the reasons why this healthy lifestyle is important, but share with them what is healthy for you and what your "why" is. Share with them what made you want to make such a family change, and how you personally see the same theme.

The children will already see that the change is happening in you. There will be less resistance, because you started the process of change two weeks ago. Once you have shared your goals with all your family members, you should create a shared vision in which all members of the family participate.

Sit together in the living room—or wherever you have a comfortable place to sit—and raise ideas together. Ask them how they see your goal. Hear their opinion about your goal, what they think about it, whether they think there are other things to add to it, or whether it is worth changing to a more accurate goal. Do they have their own goals they would like to reach? After the whole family has joined the same cause, it is time to start taking action. Each member of the family should try to come up with ideas that will help the whole family achieve the goal.

Of course, you will write down all the ideas that the whole family has, and each week you will work on one action. And, within a few weeks, you will do more and more of those small actions that gradually accumulate over time to one big change. Graduality is a very important tool for the transition to be easy and pleasant for all members of the family, and everyone can acclimatize to the new way you are aiming.

The family as a tribe

A sense of belonging is a basic and existential necessity of man. A human is a social being; from the moment of birth and throughout his life he aspires to belong.

A child who develops a belief that she belongs, that she has a place, that her parents love her, even if she is not successful and not perfect, will feel that way everywhere. She will grow up to be a self-confident person, a person who accepts herself as she is, and feels good about herself in many areas. She will not be busy proving herself, won't constantly be looking for certifications that she is fine, and she can direct her energies to realizing her unique destiny in the world.

A child who feels that he belongs and feels valuable is a child who feels good and, therefore, behaves well. A sense of belonging is not something to be won, but something to believe in. A child who feels that he has no place, will devote his energy to finding a place. Instead of contributing, he will focus on himself. When the sense of belonging of the child decreases, he acts to achieve it, often by resistance. The child's resistance is directed not at the parent but at the need for a sense of belonging. Children adopt behavioral strategies that will give them a high sense of belonging.

"All for one and one for all, united we stand divided we fall." - *Alexandre Dumas*

Let your child feel they belong

- *Create an atmosphere of acceptance* - when raising ideas, try to share your decisions with your children. Let them come up with ideas of their own and get their share of love and enthusiasm. It provides a good and important feeling for the development of their self-image.

- *Choosing from two options* - the sense of choice develops a sense of self-control, which strengthens self-esteem and the desire for cooperation. When children feel that they have a certain choice, they become partners and for less resistance. Giving them a choice makes them feel that they are treated as adults, and this feeling develops a higher self-image.

- *Responsibility* - taking responsibility is a value that needs to be taught to children from a very young age. It starts with the smallest things: returning the games to the drawer, doing homework, arranging their bag for school, etc. Even with food, a child learns the concept of "taking responsibility." In the future, the child will take responsibility for himself and his body, and thereby make sure that his diet is healthy and balanced. Children need diversity and want to experiment with many different things. Do not be fixed in the work or task you give the children. Make it possible to diversify and exchange as many roles as possible.

- *Share the child* - give him the opportunity to learn from you and share it with the actions you do. Beyond the fact that the child will begin to feel more meaningful, he will be able to learn from you more and more, whether it's how you cook or how you shop. The child will learn how to make the right choices later on his own.

Determination and perseverance

One of the most important elements in achieving goals and self-fulfillment in both children and adults is determination and perseverance. Talent is not enough. It can really help at the beginning, but talent is a small coefficient compared to persistence, investment, and passion. A person who has the discipline will not only be good at it, they could become excellent and beyond. But, why does it matter so much? Why does passion have so much of an impact on the outcome? A person who enjoys doing what he wants to achieve will have a much easier time investing in the same field. In addition, it is very important to invest outside of the mandatory timeframe that is allocated to the same action and that is when it comes from the child, and he wants to do it.

The power of persistence outside the mandatory timeframe

We will take two twin boys, both of whom are identical in their level in basketball and chess, are very talented in both fields, but each has their own interest. One is interested in chess, and the other is interested in basketball. It is reasonable to assume that each of them will spend more time in their own area of interest, even though they both started in the same situation, both of which were equal, despite the fact that both of them continued to deal in both areas simultaneously.

The result is that one of them will become an excellent basketball player and a good chess player and the other will become a great chess player and a good basketball player. The only difference between them was that while we were out of the time that was fixed, each child accumulated hours and hours of experience and that would differentiate him from a good player to an excellent one.

Assimilation of determination and perseverance

Let your child strengthen what they are good at. If he is very interested in basketball, then help him strengthen his passion and give him all the help you can. You cannot *make* a person develop a passion in something that he does not care about or develop a strong desire for success in a particular field, without interest. Help them develop the areas they are passionate about.

Let your child express the uniqueness that comes with her to the world. It may be that the parent has a desire for their child to do something like become a doctor or a basketball player, etc. But, as long as it is not burning in the child, there is no reason to push her. One of the biggest mistakes one can make is to let the child continue to do what she does not like and does not show any interest in. The child will continue to do what the parent wants just to please them. A child who has become an adult who only does what others want can hurt herself during her life and hurt her ability to listen to herself and realize the things she wants in life, because she has learned that she must always please her parents and those around her to be satisfied.

So, should he be allowed to do only what he loves and abandon the rest?

No, he has to do what he does not like, and it will have a very big impact on his personality in the future with coping with different situations and delaying gratification—you have to find the balance between the two worlds.

A child who is good in any field and likes to do it, whether it is basketball, music, or any other field, and he persists in it and succeeds in it, will build a sense of ability and faith in himself and his abilities in the field he loves. The feeling will generally exist in him and will affect many other areas of his life, and it will create positive improvements in many other areas that will lead to improved results. It is possible that the child will move from field to field until he finds his passion, and that is excellent.

The role of parents is to encourage desire

It can be in any field that the child chooses. For example, you'll put a basket in your backyard, or go to a basketball court every day or twice a week to work on the technique.

Give the child the resources to flourish so that he will discover his destiny, help him find his interests and what inspires him in that desire, and encourage him and give him the resources he needs. In exploring these new places, it will be much easier for him to discover new places within his inner and outer world.

The power of deferring gratification

So, what do we know about postponing gratification?
Studies that have been published for decades that examined the development of children have found that there are two main important characteristics related to success in life: one is rejection of gratification, and the other is persistence. If we think about it for a second, the same attributes are related to each other so that the second one will be required.

Emotional development and rejection of gratification

Emotional regulation and rejection of gratification - the ability to relinquish immediate reward and the strong desire to gain immediate reward. A parent who educates his children in such a way that he meets his child's demands immediately, does not prepare his children for real life. He creates the opposite effect and teaches his child a virtual reality. In other words, he makes his children think that in the real world everything happens right now and at that moment according to how he wants and when he wants. And, as most of us know, the world does not give everything at once, and sometimes things take time.

What will the child experience when he hears "No!" for the first time in his life? It is likely that he will feel great frustration and helplessness and even a decline in his self-confidence, and that situation will greatly affect him. A person's ability to postpone gratification is a very important trait for dealing with different situations in life from proper nutrition to business. Delaying satisfaction has a great impact on childhood and adult life. A child who grows up with a high ability to reject gratification will have a much better future.

The marshmallow experiment

In the 1960s, an experiment was conducted at Stanford University by researcher Walter Michelle, a study that can be found in his famously named Marshmallow Experiment. This experiment was conducted on children aged two to four.

How was the experiment conducted?
Each child in turn entered an empty room and sat down on a chair. On the table in front of them lay a lone marshmallow. The experimenter explained to the child that he would leave the room for a while, and the child had a choice. The child could eat the one marshmallow, or, if he waited until the experimenter returned, they would get two marshmallows instead of just one.

The results were interesting. It turned out that two out of three children could not resist eating the one marshmallow. Some could not hold back for more than a few seconds after the experimenter left the room. In contrast, one-third of the children held back, some with great difficulty, and strained not to be tempted to eat the one marshmallow. The children smudged, fingered, and stared at the one marshmallow, but they did not eat it prematurely. They waited for the experimenter to return so they could eat two marshmallows.

It's a real experience to watch this experiment.

You are welcome to watch the video at:

www.omgoverweight.com/marshmallow

But this is not the end of the experiment. The interesting part is that they went to check on the condition of these children after fourteen years.

The researchers returned to the children who had grown up in the meantime and were about to graduate from high school. The revelations were fascinating. It turned out that of the group of children who managed to postpone satisfactions, a very high percentage showed more developed social and educational abilities than the group of children who did not restrain themselves and ate the one marshmallow ahead of time. In addition, the children who managed to delay gratification grew up to be adults who coped better with frustration and stress.

This study clearly shows the critical importance of learning to postpone gratification from a very young age. The experiment teaches us, as parents, that saying 'no' to a toddler or a child does not only achieve a specific and short-term goal, such as not eating candy, but it is most significant to the future temptation and success of our children.

As always, a personal example in front of the children is helpful. The child also learns from his parents how to cope with postponing gratification in eating and other issues in life.

Building a rejection of gratification

- Distraction - What needs to be done is to distract the child from the ice cream with the elegance of the ice cream. You can suggest that you do anything else—listen to a story, sing songs, dance, or play a game. Do whatever it takes to make him forget that you talked about ice cream. In the world of ADHD, it can be very easy. It must be remembered that this is only a rejection, not a refusal. Eventually, every child will remember that he did not get the ice cream he wanted.

- Expanding the timeframe, depending on the child's age and level of development, it is possible to simply extend the time from the moment the request was made, until later on. It can be an hour, two hours, an entire day, or even weeks.

- Building a postponement of gratification with the Internet - When a game is ordered off the Internet for your child, there is a delay between when you ordered the game for them and when they receive it in a few days. So, the child knows that the game is on the way to him, but he will have to deal with the "difficulty" of waiting until it finally reaches him.

Let him manage on his own

First, let the child try to do what he asked help for. There is no need to run straight to it and do what he asked. For example, if your child asked you to help him solve something in his homework—even though he had not even opened the notebook or tried on his own—it is very important that you tell him and explain to him that he has to start alone and see how he manages on his own. Of course, there is no need to ignore the child's request and not give him any attention. In the end, ignoring is not a rejection of gratification, but one must not respond directly to every request by your child. Give him the opportunity to solve the problem himself. This can be very helpful to your child. In addition to helping build gratification, it creates a feeling of competence in the child.

Another example is when you are busy with something else and the child asks for your help. You do not always have to help him. You can tell him that you have heard his request, and that you are finishing a few things. But, in the meantime, he can try to solve the problem on his own. Or, once you're done, you'll go to him and go through it together to see how he did it, or if he still needs help.

Depending on your child's age and level of understanding, you can tell him that you believe in him and that you think he can do it alone (if possible) or that he can wait for you. Be patient and give a personal example. If the child asks again and again like a child does, try to keep him cool and patient. Explain to him that you will be able to help him in a few minutes. If you do this and explain it to the child and he still doesn't stop nagging you, you can simply ignore his actions without feeling any anger, and then turn to him when you're finished.

It is very important that you give positive feedback if the child can wait patiently until you have approached him. Encourage him and give him positive reinforcement. It is very important to build a sense of success in the child and give the child the desire to postpone the satisfaction once again, because he knows that he will be rewarded for it. Symbolic gifts can also be used as a success in deferring satisfaction, such as a sticker or a common game that he loves. It is very important to understand that food and sweets are not a good solution to a symbolic gift. I will explain this during the part of the book on nutrition.

Setting boundaries

Should boundaries be set? Maybe you should just let the child do what he wants?

It is not clear to every parent why boundaries are needed in raising children, and in life in general. The emphasis on a child's need for love and acceptance has resulted in unprecedented forgiveness and responsiveness to the child's demands. Ultimately, the goal of all parents is to let the children grow up happy but, sometimes, with all this love, a parent can deprive their children of one of the most basic things—boundaries.

A child who is exposed to conflicts during her life will help further her development. A child who is shown clear boundaries and is exposed to these confrontations will experience confidence because she knows that there are those who are watching over her. Someone sees her and cares for her. A show of weakness in front of the child creates the exact opposite result. It undermines the child's confidence, and she does not have the knowledge that she has someone to trust and care for her. It is very important to give the child the feeling that she has someone to trust. By setting clear boundaries, the parent defines expectations for the child and, of course, the parent must continue to serve as a personal example. One cannot expect the child to perform something that the parent does not do.

Studies completed in the 1980s showed that children growing up in permissive education systems are characterized by high levels of violence, dropouts, drug abuse, delinquency, and sexual promiscuity. These children were characterized with a particularly low self-image.

A self-image develops not only through hugs, but also when a parent tells the crying child who is going into kindergarten, "You'll stay in the garden, and I'll pick you up at the end of the day. I love you and I know you want me to stay with you, but you have to stay in the garden, and you have to deal with it." Of course, I'm not talking about the very first day of kindergarten.

Permissiveness, indulgence, and overprotection create the same effect as humiliation. What does this mean? Preventing the child from experiencing his own power and the feeling that he is capable on his own can create many negative effects in the child, as a child and during their adult life. They can grow up feeling that you always feel sorry for them, that they deserve everything and it may even develop a sense of incompetence. In the event that the parent does not use any boundaries, he teaches the child to pity himself and that can create a feeling in the child that life owes him something, and anything he wants he should receive right then!

The same issue causes the problem of delaying gratification. Once the child grows up and becomes an adult, it can create a great conflict between the way he sees real life.

When a parent sets a boundary for a child, the child will naturally examine the parent's boundary and even do exactly the opposite of what the parent has asked of him.

If the parent asks him not to eat in the living room, he will, of course, go and eat in the living room. He will try everything to stay in the living room and eat there, and he will find a thousand and one reasons why he should eat in the living room. He will ask again and again, even though you explained it to him, and it seemed that he understood very well why he shouldn't eat in the living room. This is where the subject of educating rejection of satisfactions comes into play. The parent wants to teach his child that this is the limit at home and that action will cause the child to develop qualities of gratification. So, the role of the parent is that he will have to help his child overcome their desire and their demands and obey the rules, although it may be less pleasant for them.

Requirements for setting boundaries
- *The parent needs to know what the limit is* - The child needs to know what the limit is, and the parent needs to be aware of what their limits are—what they think is fine and what is not. Once the parent knows exactly what they want, they can set a clear and precise boundary for the child.
- *Coordination between the two parents* - It is very important that there be coordination between the parents. A lack of coordination prevents the creation of boundaries and, whenever the child wants to break a boundary, he will go to the other

parent, because he did not like the answer of the first parent. There must be full synchronization and cooperation between the two parents.

- *Personal example and setting boundaries* - Do not expect your children to do something that you do not do. In the end, children learn a lot by watching a parent and acting in imitation. If you tell them something, but you do exactly the opposite, do not expect too much.

- *Consistency* – Parents need to be consistent in their decisions and stand by each other. A child will try to check the boundaries again and again. What the child does is check your consistency about the limit you set. She checks how much you stand behind what you say. Each child has her own personality. There are children who will understand the boundary very quickly, and there are children who will try to stretch the boundary. Once there is no consistency, the child will see the breach in the boundary, and it will simply not be possible to build a clear boundary.

- *Perseverance* - The moment you decide what the limit is, you need to stick to it. If you change your mind every moment, you will be influenced by your child, and she will never experience what a limit is.

- *A clear boundary* - You need to set a clear boundary. It may not be easy at first, if it means that the child has left the bedroom twenty times, and you have to put him back in bed twenty times. But, do it until he stays in bed, and he accepts your limit.

- *Definitely* - Did you know that ninety percent of the communication between people is transmitted through the subconscious, such as body language, body posture, tone of voice, etc.? Only about ten percent of our communications are transmitted through our conscious mind.

This means that the message will be conveyed in a clear and precise manner. There must be a correspondence between the way you say things and the way you express them. For example, if you tell the child to go back to bed and then you smile or laugh every time he gets out of bed, you didn't create a clear boundary, and the child noticed it. You must really mean what you say and stand behind what you say. Your words represent only ten percent of the communication, and the child sees the ninety percent that completely contradicts what you say. Pay attention to your tone of voice, to your body language, and to the energy that comes with you when you are setting a limit.

- *Practical tone of voice and respect* – Quite often, when parents set limits, they lose their temper and speak unpleasantly to their children. And, that does not contribute to their learning.
- *Explain* - the familiar question from all children is **why**?
Never answer: because I said so!

You are working out your ability to teach the child about the situation. For the child to understand what your intention was to the thing you said or did, it is very important to explain this to him in parallel to the situation, and not in retrospect. Once it is clear to the child why you responded as you did, it will be easier for him to understand why you chose to act the way you did.

You can see beautiful examples on the TV program, *Supernanny*, and the power of persistence and setting boundaries. How many children change once they see that there is a slightly more authoritative figure who knows what she wants and stands behind her statements?

Every failure is a source of growth

From the moment a person came to life, he began to experience failures. We experienced failures. Like babies who tried to walk and fell, we failed every time. As children, we could not read and write and, each time, we failed again. So, it seems that failure is natural and that it is a normal part of a person's development and progress. So, the question is whether there is such a thing as *failure*?

I believe not. There is such a thing as learning, and learning comes from growth. A person cannot succeed if he cannot experience failures during his life, and he avoids those failures over and over again. If you learn from "failure" then it is no longer considered a failure.

So, what is failure?
Failure is an interpretation. It's a way of looking at things. Say we take two kids and let them run in a race, and both of them get a low score. One child will understand that he is bad, and not good at it, and will not do it again. The other child will take that temporary failure and understand that he needs to improve in order to be better. So, the next time he does the same test, he will come prepared, and he will have a much better result. So, what we understand

from that is that failure is subjective in accordance with the interpretation of how a person or a child perceives himself in relation to that situation.

Failures in children's lives

A child with high self-confidence will take the failure to a place of learning and development and improve for the next time; they see it only as a milestone. A child of low self-confidence will take the same failure as something personal and will see himself as a failure. If he got a failing score in the test, then he's a failure. The child connects himself directly to the result and does not see the separateness.

It is important that you help your children make the distinction between the outcome they get and the way they perceive themselves. Give them the tools to recognize that failure is part of learning.

As an inventor, Edison made 1,000 unsuccessful attempts at inventing the light bulb.

When a reporter asked, "How did it feel to fail 1,000 times?"

Edison replied, "I didn't fail 1,000 times. The light bulb was an invention with 1,000 steps."

Evaluation based on investment and effort rather than outcome

As I described in the previous section, a child who sees himself as identifying with the result he has received for the purpose fails in mathematics and sees himself as a failure. First grade scores the children according to grades, which can harm the self-confidence of the child and they can see themselves as unsuccessful or unwise.

So, what can the parent do?

The role of the parent is not to criticize the score or the school that does the scoring. The role of the parent is to assess the level of investment or lack of investment of the child. Explain to the children that, despite the results of the test, they are already successful. And, their success depends on what they do, even if it is currently a challenging area for them. They can become very good in the same field with an additional investment of their time and a dedication to the task. The result is not really important, they just need to spend more time on it and do their best every time. You will teach them that they are responsible for their ability to succeed, and they have all the capabilities to reach any outcome they choose to reach.

Separation between the child and the action

Is there really such a thing as bad children or problematic children?
The child himself is naturally good, and there is no child whose purpose is to do a bad or evil act, or to get his parent out of his head, although sometimes it can look like this. If he has chosen to do something, it is reasonable to assume that he has a whole story behind him. It can be attention-grabbing, emotional deprivation, a boundary

128

check, or simply naive mischief. The way he behaves can be problematic, or the act he did was not good. It is very important to note that you do not combine the same action that the child has made with the child himself. The child is not bad; the action was bad.

For example, a parent who says to his child, "You are a bad boy!" The moment they criticize him and not what he did, he will learn nothing from it. And, instead of criticizing his behavior, this statement criticizes the child as if he were the act itself.

Words have a lot of power. So, pay attention to what words you use in front of your children and the way you choose to express what you have to say. You can say that this behavior is behavior that you do not like, etc. And that's why he came into the room. What this sentence tells the child is that he did not behave well and, on the other hand, he was not told that he was a bad boy. He was told that the action he had done was wrong.

Compliment mainly on actions

Compliment him not only on the grade he received but on the things he did to get the score. He studied and did homework in preparation for the test, listened to lessons, searched, etc. The result he received is not really important; always remember to reinforce the actions taken to achieve the result. The "result" is just a number.

How is it possible to improve a result?
The only way is to change or improve the actions that went before.

Reinforcing actions - Tell her she was good for investing time in her studies and for the hours she spent after school working on homework. Tell her she was ready for the test because she practiced the material.

Reinforcing Characteristics – Tell her you are so proud of her for her perseverance, her determination, and how motivated she was to succeed, etc.

Positive feedback
It is important for children to give themselves positive feedback.

A child who is able to strengthen himself on his successes will need less reinforcement from the environment in the future, because his inner world is stable enough. On the other hand, children with low self-esteem will be affected mainly by the environment and feedback they will receive for each action they take. The child must be given a message that the strengths are in him and the successes are his. Although there are people who will not always believe in everything he does, because they do not believe they can do it themselves, he should believe in himself. Once he believes in himself, he will know he could really do it. Help him build his faith in himself and the determination that there is nothing to resist.

The little frog

There was a group of tiny frogs who decided to organize a running competition. The goal was to reach the top of a very tall tower. A large crowd gathered around the tower to see the competition and encourage the competitors. The competition began, and the truth was that no one in the audience really believed that the tiny frogs would reach the top of the tower.

There were cries such as, "It's too hard," "They'll never get to the top," or "They're not going to succeed; the tower is too high!" And it happened that, during the climb, the little frogs began to collapse. One tiny frog continued to climb higher and higher at an accelerated pace, and the crowd continued to shout, "It's too hard! No one will succeed!" More tiny frogs got tired and gave up, and only one frog continued to rise higher and higher.

That frog would not give up. Eventually, all the frogs gave up and stopped climbing the tower except for one tiny frog, that, after a lot of effort, was the only one to reach the top of the tower. All the other tiny frogs wanted to know how this little frog had succeeded. How was she the only one who could do this of all the strong and experienced frogs?

The little frog did not answer.

The other frogs asked her again, "What was your secret? How did you do it?"

The frog still did not answer.

Then they remembered that this little frog was deaf.

This story is told to teach us about how much influence the environment has on us, and the many beliefs that people have about themselves and throw at us. Because they don't think they can, they don't think the rest of us can. You need to develop in your child the knowledge that they are capable and able to accomplish whatever they desire. And they do not have to listen to those voices that do not believe. The only person they need to believe in ... is themselves!

Ways to strengthen self-belief

Encourage children to praise themselves: "I am successful." "I am strong." "I am beautiful." This action does not cause narcissism or arrogance. Because the child does not say, "I am the best," "I am the strongest," or "I am the most successful." They simply put him in a place where he does not compare himself to anyone, and he simply states a fact. Saying this fact helps him to establish his belief in himself and belief in what he can do and achieve. Strong self-belief has a great influence on the confidence that a child will have in life, so help him establish it. You can do this practice in front of the mirror with your child. Tell him to look himself in the mirror, and then tell him to say something about himself after you say something about yourself.

Then you start saying the positive reinforcements like, "I'm smart" and then the child comes back with, "I'm successful." You can do this as many times as you like, and you should adopt it as a daily ritual at the end of each day.

It is very important to listen to your children and talk to them to see what their thinking patterns are, what they have in mind about themselves, and their abilities. Once you recognize that a child has a limiting belief about herself or thinks she is unable to do something, you can help her make the change to a better way of thinking and change it into strong thinking.

You can go over the part we talked about changing thinking patterns and deepening the steps needed to help your children change their beliefs about themselves.

Constructive criticism

Criticism is one of the ways to educate and teach children to act correctly. The problem is that if you do not do it in the right way, the criticism can hurt. You can treat the criticism as a gift that you want to give your children. The problem is that, in general, not everyone is happy to receive the gift of criticism. Even adults are not always interested in hearing criticism, even if its goal is positive. The goal of the parent is to pass the review without the child realizing that it is criticism. Children are very sensitive, and if they do not perform the check correctly, then the same goal that was to help them improve the situation only makes it worse.

Tips for constructive criticism

- Perform the criticism in a positive manner and come to the situation as calmly as possible.
- Sometimes, a later critique is more effective than a critique of the moment. If a child did something that really irritated a parent, it would be very difficult for the parent, at that moment, to react to the situation in a balanced way, and in the way that the parent would not be too angry.
- It is very important to praise the child before reaching the stage of criticism. The praise stage is very important and effective. It helps to lower defenses and allows criticism to be absorbed in a much lighter and more effective way.

The way to criticize has great power and will allow your child to absorb what you are saying without directly defending herself and doing exactly the opposite of what you are asking for. Of course, there are cases where the parent will have to be more assertive in some cases.

Say only the truth

Intuition - Intuition is the ability to decode messages and situations without voluntary thinking. You may intuitively know the answer, or it may come instantly or suddenly to you. You may get a gut feeling, or a very common female intuition about the subject.

Did you have a bad gut feeling about something and you were right about it? That was your intuition! People think that the signs will be clear as the sun. The truth is that the signals of intuition do not shout. They whisper very weakly. Those who can control their intuition are women who are more connected to their feelings.

Apart from women, children are also very attached to their intuition. That is why it is very important not to lie to your children!

You don't have to say a single word for the child to feel what you really think. Children are not mind readers, or there would be such chaos. But it's pretty close. Children can sense whether you are lying to them or if you are telling the truth. If you have complimented the child on something he did, and you real didn't mean it, then there is a good chance that he will notice it, because they are very attentive to their feelings and their intuition. If there is a contrast between what is said and the child's inner feelings, it will cause the child to feel distrust of what he has been told. It can even create a crisis of trust with the parents, because the parents lied to him and did not tell the truth.

Children have an amazing ability to read a situation. An adult accumulates a wealth of experiences and events in the course of a life that sometimes may lead to immunity to those sensations, which leads to a person being less attentive to the internal thinking, and they act more from the head than from the heart.

The important things to avoid are:

- *Do not tease the child or call him names-* either in public or at home, if the child is overweight. A parent should not tease about fat, weight, or food, nor laugh at the child! Remember, it is likely that the child is not happy about the situation he is in, and if he notices that he is an exception to those around him, then he does not like it. In addition, it may be that in school they mock the child with nicknames. Think about how it may make your child feel. Your intention may be completely different, but what the child feels about that word will not necessarily make him feel good about it, and those words can even make matters worse. In addition, the moment you define the child as obese, this can put the child in the sense that it is the tortoise, and that's who he is, and that he cannot do anything about it.
- *Do not blame -* A parent should not say to the child, "Are you eating sweets again?" or "How much food do you eat?"
  The parent first needs to check with himself on a number of things. Is he part of the process the child is going through? Did the parent stop buying sweets and give the child healthy alternatives? You cannot demand something from the child if he does not have the tools to do it.

In addition, the parent should be a role model. If they do not eat healthy foods, their child will not either. It doesn't matter if you are a proper weight and you do not have to lose weight. The parent should be a role model. In addition, every time the parent blames the child, it makes the child feel that the parent is not accepting the child as he is and that he has no place to belong. It creates the opposite situation if the child did something that he "should not do." It is important to respond moderately, and if necessary, do not react at the moment. Wait until later. And don't react with strangers around. Only do it at home and in front of the immediate family where the child will feel comfortable.

- *Do not compare* - Many parents compare their child to another child to make it clear to the child what they have done wrong. But, this is a very problematic way, which can greatly harm the child's self-confidence. The very fact that you put the child in a position that is equal to another person, you are telling him he is not good enough. It is important to understand that every person is an individual and unique. A similar thing happens in many cases when there are brothers or sisters at home and the parent tries to explain to the child how to behave by using an example of a brother or sister who behaved in the right way.
A common sentence used by parents: "Why do you behave like that? Look at your brother and how beautifully he behaves." This message has a negative impact on the child's self-confidence and, in addition, can create a distance between the brothers. This can create the exact opposite

situation whose purpose was to teach the child what is right to do. However, once the child sees that he cannot compete against his brother, he may choose to be "the bad boy."

That's why it's so important to never compare your child to their brothers or sisters, or anyone else! You should not compare two children, and you should not compare two people. Everyone is an entity unto itself, and they are born with their own personality traits, abilities, and skills.

Chapter 4:
Nutrition

The overall picture

One of the most important issues we talk about is obesity in the world, as we have already understood that the change will last for a long time, we need to look at the overall picture. Changing nutrition will not be enough to create a long-term change. So, the first parts of this book talk about the body and the mind, and emotional and environmental habits.

Nutrition is the main thing that leads to weight loss but, on the other hand, it is still the hardest part. Most of our nutritional habits are built during childhood. The child learns and receives from his parents the habits that develop into adulthood. So, it is very important to build healthy eating habits in children as young as possible.

Today's diet

We cannot ignore the culture of fast food. In the past, there was no fast food and people didn't have to worry about what they ate. Now, we can eat Japanese, Indian, Chinese, Mediterranean, or Italian food all within thirty minutes of pressing the order key on our mobile phone. Beyond the fact that food has become so accessible, a lot of ingredients are added to it that are not really necessary.

When was the last time you had a look at a list of ingredients of the things you buy?

If you check the ingredients in your bread, you will discover that there are five other ingredients that you have no idea what they are and which are completely unnecessary. These additives aim to improve the taste and smell of the food and extend their shelf life.

Healthy and balanced diet

A balanced diet can have a significant impact on the lives of your children. Here are some examples:

- Preventing the tendency to obesity—which is affected, among other things, by the number of fat cells. The production of fat cells occurs until the teen years. After this age, obesity (or weight loss) is actually the expansion (or reduction) of existing fat cells. The larger the amount of fat cells created during this period, the greater the tendency for obesity in the future.
- The amount of muscle cells is also strongly affected during childhood
- Building an effective immune system for disease prevention and reducing the potential for adult diabetes
- Normal nervous system activity that affects the speed and accuracy of reactions to situations because nerves and nerve cells are created during this period and do not regenerate afterwards
- Realizing the potential for development and growth of the body
- Build strong skeletal bones and strong teeth
- Proper nutrition helps to significantly alleviate ADHD and concentration in general

How is being overweight caused?

"More calories coming in than are exported causes weight problems and obesity."

If everyone understands what the problem is causing people to get fat, why do people keep getting fat?

Today more than ever, people are obsessed with calories.

Maybe it's a matter of genetics?
If we go back a few years, people were not as fat as today, and they weren't as sick as today.

Medicine has helped us to extend the number of years that a person lives but, on the other hand, the quality of those years is poor. The world tries to blame behavior itself, and they say it is a matter of willpower. That is true, but it is not the only element. There are things that make it difficult for a person to make the right decision and persist. If it was so simple, everyone would do it and keep their weight down over time. In the first part of this book in the body and mind section, we learned that emotional eating compensates people for other inadequacies. For them, in this part of the book, we will learn what happens in the brain and human body biochemically, what causes children to eat more, what the implications are of certain foods, and what the most problematic components are that have taken over our diet.

What makes us want to eat?

We eat for one reason—our brain tells us to eat. What does that mean? It is not the person who decides consciously when to eat. The person chooses what to put in a cake or a cookie, but what happens before that is the brain telling the person to put the food in their mouth. A number of chemical changes activate the mechanism of hunger spread by their brain and the result is "I'm hungry; I have to eat."

There are biochemical changes that happen all the time in the body that affect the feeling of hunger. Hunger can be caused by different situations such as stress, emotional compensation, or even a lack of sleep. There is also great importance on the type of food that a person puts into their body. Some foods can harm your judgment or your decisions.

The connection between rewards, satisfaction, addictions, and being overweight

The biochemical *sense of reward* causes a dopamine secretion, and a *sense of satisfaction* causes the secretion of serotonin.

Each of these hormones activates areas of the brain that trigger emotions. Each of them has its own region and its connections and has a different effect on the emotions on the mind and body.

What are the differences?

Reward - for a short period of time, holding an hour at the end, it can be motivated by a good meal.

Satisfaction - holds for a long time and even for life, for example the ceremony of awarding certificates at your son's university.

Reward - brings the person to a sense of excitement, like winning a casino game raises your excitement level and your blood pressure and pulse rise; these feelings rarely occur.

Satisfaction – happens more often, such as listening to music or watching the sea; these actions do exactly the opposite—they lower your blood pressure, slow your pulse, and put your body into a state of relaxation.

Reward - can be achieved from various drugs like caffeine, alcohol, and sugar, each of which activates the sense of reward in the brain.

Satisfaction - cannot be achieved with the help of these physical things.

Reward - is momentary, like buying or wearing clothes for the first time and, after the first time, the enthusiasm wears off .

Satisfaction - can come from giving, and the feeling will be sustained over time, such as donating money to a charity, spending time with your children, or investing time into something that is important to you.

Reward - is only yours and yours alone, and does not affect anyone else around you.

Satisfaction - affects your environment, and other people besides you who enjoy the action you did.

Reward - without attention can lead to addiction, e.g., too much food or alcohol, and obsession with certain things can cause many health problems and even death in some cases.

Satisfaction - cannot create addictions.

Dopamine and weight gain

- A person suffering from morbid obesity is above the healthy range of dopamine. In addition to that, if a person is stressed, it will be even worse. Dopamine causes confusion. Leptin neurons generally oppose and balance dopamine, but if a person is in a state of morbid obesity, they do not object. They just do not work.

- Drugs and addictions change the balance of dopamine receptors, which causes a situation where the feeling is not satisfied. As long as dopamine remains high, a person will have to eat again and again in order to achieve the same sense of reward. People who are in a state of morbid obesity have 30-40 percent fewer dopamine receptors.

- Dopamine is only the trigger. It is produced initially in the first thrill, before consumption, when you have the desire to eat something that you really crave. This is the moment when dopamine is excreted. The experience does not end until the end of consumption or the act that includes the same sense of euphoria and pleasure that causes an additional secretion of chemicals, which affects the hypothalamus, which is a region of the brain that controls the area of emotions and feelings.

Just as betting one time will not turn a person into a gambler, and just as one drug experiment will not turn a person into a drug addict, so it is with sugar. You will not become addicted to sugar and other carbohydrates after one or two tastes. But, on the other hand, continually eating sugar and carbohydrates will create an addiction, and you will crave them and want more and more.

When should you start worrying?

When you see that a child is not satisfied with the same consumption of the same foods over and over again, that he does not achieve the same sense of reward and does not settle for the experiential result of it, then you should start worrying.

These situations can indicate a situation in which the child or adult is exposed to dopamine exposure or decreased dopamine receptors. This leaves the person in a constant state of dissatisfaction and a desire for further consumption. This can lead to increased consumption, which needs to increase from time to time in order to achieve the same sense of experience, and this ultimately leads to addiction.

Why do we like sweet-tasting foods?

Evolution- babies are completely instinctive, showing a clear preference for sweet mother's milk, over other non-sweet drinks. The evolutionary reason: sweet food contains sugar and sugar is a source of available energy. So, from a survival point of view, the attraction to sweet food will ensure a supply of calories, which, in ancient times, were not as readily available as today.

Exposure at a young age- small children learn what the "right" taste of food is when exposed to various foods. Studies have shown that children who have become accustomed to eating sugary foods will prefer sweeter foods, even as adults. That is, the level of sweetness they will like will be high. Studies have found that if children consume more fruit, it will lower their sweetness requirements. They learn that the level of sweetness in fruit is better than sweet foods like chocolate cake.

Behaviorally - Breastfeeding provides not only the baby's growing needs, but also their emotional needs. Suckling, and later eating, is a source of relaxation and consolation. Because mother's milk is sweet and oily, the baby learns the connection between sweet and high-fat foods and sedation and comfort. The problem is that parental comfort tends to use the mechanism of an attraction to sweets at an early age in order to encourage the child to eat. The parent sweetens foods so that the baby will eat better foods, and, at a later age, they reward the child by giving him a cookie for good behavior or for compensation and relaxation when the child cries.

All of these situations build up an unhealthy base and attitude for the child that will become more problematic over the years. Many people, as well as children, turn to sweets to soothe the need for "something," usually as a result of stress and also to get instant energy. But the quickest solution is not always ideal. As fast as blood sugar rises, it decreases, causing another need for sweet food, and so on.

What is the stress from sugar?

What caused all this hysteria about sugar? Sugar was not readily available to most people until recent years. What happened? Why are people so concerned with sugar now? And, why, specifically, do we now see the consequences of eating sugar?

Many years ago, there was no problem with sugar, because it was not as accessible as today. Exposure to sugar was very low compared to today. The problem began when the food industry began to add sugar to everything. The thing is that sugar is not part of our required nutrients.

Alcohol is not considered as one of our nutritional requirements, and we know what the consequences are of a high intake of alcohol, and how it can affect our behavior and physical state. But, are we aware enough of the consequences of an excessive consumption of sugar? How does sugar affect our body, our decisions, or our emotional state? Most of us do not drink alcohol every day. And, even if it is not in large quantities, for the reason that alcohol is not readily available, it is not suitable for consumption in most situations.

Usually, a person will consume alcohol during the evening, after he has reached the house and wants to rest or for social recreation. Sugar, on the other hand, is consumed throughout the day. It is readily available, and it can be consumed several times during the day without disturbing other activities.

The problem is that the majority of people are not aware of the high consumption of sugars, which children put into their bodies. Sugar consumption does not end with the amount of sweets or snacks given to a child that day. The problem is that today there is sugar in almost every industrial food we eat.

The difference between glucose and fructose

Glucose - The body knows how to use glucose reserves for a wide range of uses. Glucose is used as an energy source, and it is the main sugar found in the blood. It is the preferred substance of the brain and muscles, meaning glucose is used as renewable energy and is available to all parts of the body. Red blood cells can only use glucose as energy. When a person puts glucose into his body, the body breaks it down with insulin.

Fructose - It is the worst sugar, and it has the least glycemic value. Fructose is stored only in the liver, weighs heavily on it, and is a major factor in insulin immunity. It does not break down in the blood and no other organ can use it. Fructose is found in fruits, and you cannot reach high levels of fructose from eating only fruits. The problem is that fructose is found in almost all types of industrial foods, which leads to an increased consumption, and, in most cases, without people knowing about it.

One of the reasons that fructose is used as a sweetener is because it is very cheap.

Where is the sugar hiding?

There are many names for those sugars that appear on the packaging that will make it difficult for the customer to recognize that it is sugar, which means that we do not know how much sugar we are putting into our bodies. Before you buy a packaged product, look at the label on the product to see if it contains sugar (sugar can hide under many names).

Sugar substitutes

People think that sugar substitutes are better than regular sugar, but the opposite is true. Although the caloric value is very low, and sometimes even reaches zero, is it just the calories that make us fat? Or is the insulin level important in the blood?

Sugar substitutes not only increase insulin levels in the blood, they sometimes raise the levels more than normal sugar does.

This includes the "natural" sweeteners like stevia. These sweeteners not only cause an increase in insulin that interferes with blood sugar absorption and causes liver overload, they also cause cravings and a desire for sweetness like regular sugar does. These sweeteners can sometimes taste a few times sweeter than sucrose, for example, while stevia powder tastes 200 to 300 times sweeter than regular sugar.

The question is, if you advertise all the diet drinks as diet drinks, it should mean that the person who consumes them should lose weight. However, it's not like that. If you think about it for a second, have you ever heard of someone losing weight because they drank diet drinks?

If you list some foods or drinks as "diet," it doesn't mean that it's any better. They may not use sucrose, and they may use other sweeteners with low calories, but that doesn't mean it's any better. The same "diet" drinks still cause a significant increase in insulin levels in the blood due to those sweeteners.

The 56 Most Common Names for Sugar

1 – 3

1. Sugar/Sucrose

2. High-Fructose Corn Syrup (HFCS)

   - HFCS 55: This is the most common type of HFCS. It contains 55% fructose and 45% glucose, which makes it similar to sucrose in composition.
   - HFCS 90: This form contains 90% fructose.

3. Agave Nectar

4 – 37: Other Sugars with Glucose and Fructose

4. Beet sugar
5. Blackstrap molasses
6. Brown sugar
7. Buttered syrup
8. Cane juice crystals
9. Cane sugar
10. Caramel
11. Carob syrup
12. Castor sugar
13. Coconut sugar
14. Confectioner's sugar (powdered sugar)
15. Date sugar

16. Demerara sugar
17. Evaporated cane juice
18. Florida crystals
19. Fruit juice
20. Fruit juice concentrate
21. Golden sugar
22. Golden syrup
23. Grape sugar
24. Honey
25. Icing sugar
26. Invert sugar
27. Maple syrup
28. Molasses
29. Muscovado sugar
30. Panela sugar
31. Raw sugar
32. Refiner's syrup
33. Sorghum syrup
34. Sucanat
35. Treacle sugar
36. Turbinado sugar
37. Yellow sugar

38 – 52: Sugars with Glucose
38. Barley malt
39. Brown rice syrup
40. Corn syrup
41. Corn syrup solids
42. Dextrin
43. Dextrose
44. Diastatic malt
45. Ethyl maltol

46. Glucose
47. Glucose solids
48. Lactose
49. Malt syrup
50. Maltodextrin
51. Maltose
52. Rice syrup

53 – 54: Sugars with Fructose Only
53. Crystalline fructose
54. Fructose

55 – 56: Other Sugars
55. D-ribose
56. Galactose

Insulin

What is insulin?

Insulin is produced in our body by an organ called the pancreas. Insulin is a hormone produced by the endocrine part of the pancreas. This part of the pancreas is called the Langerhans, and it consists of five different types of cells that are differentiated by the type of hormone they produce. The insulin hormone is secreted by cells called beta cells directly into the bloodstream. Insulin moves through the bloodstream and reaches the tissues where it works. Insulin is sometimes referred to as the "satiety hormone," because its normal blood levels rise after a meal—when blood sugar rises. The main role of insulin is to regulate your blood sugar level and make sure it is not too high.

Insulin and obesity

The frequency at which we put food into our mouths is determined by two centers in the brain: the hunger center and the center of satiety. The two centers work in direct contact with the stomach, and when it fills up, it transmits to the brain that it has received what it needs. The two factors are balanced by one center suppressing the other, and vice versa. When there is a state of insulin resistance, the cells are hungry for sugar, and the hunger mechanism works too much.

So, as long as insulin is secreted into the blood, in terms of the brain, it is in a state of lack of energy and, in such a situation, has no interest in increasing metabolism and wasting energy. On the contrary, it causes the body to slow down its actions in order to conserve energy. The sugar does not stabilize back to a balanced state; it falls below the normal level, causing the hunger to return.

What causes an increase in insulin levels?
To summarize, it is those foods that raise the level of insulin that cause obesity. Those foods are high in carbohydrates and sugars. The problem arises when the insulin level rises and remains high over time, which results in insulin resistance, and the body does not produce the same amount needed to balance the level of sugars in the blood, which will eventually lead to obesity.

How do you stabilize the level of insulin in the blood?
To break the cycle of high insulin levels, you have to have a low level of insulin for a period of time so that the body will get used to it and adapt to the change. Every person, before they began to suffer from obesity, had a low immunity to insulin at the beginning.

Excessive obesity and an increased immunity to insulin lead to high levels of insulin in the blood, which ultimately leads to obesity. And, not only high levels of insulin cause insulin immunity; immunity is also associated with the timing of meals, food types, and micro-nutrients. The two components are very important, but the most important element is what we eat. It is important to understand that insulin immunity is caused when there are high levels of insulin in the blood over time and not because of "peaks." This means that if most of the time the insulin levels are low and only occasionally the levels rise, the body will not produce the immunity.

What about carbohydrates?

There are two main types of carbohydrates, and it is important to make the distinction between them.

Simple carbohydrates

Simple carbohydrates are all sourced from white flour: white pasta, couscous, white rice, pita bread, and white bread.

Simple carbohydrates provide only short-term energy, like candy. They have little nutritional value, they raise blood sugar levels, and they cause a rapid increase followed by a rapid fall in blood sugar levels. They are low in fiber and can cause many undesirable symptoms, such as fatigue, lack of concentration, hyperactivity, anxiety, dizziness, blood lipids, shortness of breath, allergies, blurring of vision, weight gain, diabetes, and more.

Complex carbohydrates

Complex carbohydrates include whole grains: whole wheat bread, whole wheat flour, whole grain rice, oatmeal, lentils of various kinds, quinoa beans, sweet potatoes, etc. The release of sugar to the blood in complex carbohydrates is done slowly and does not cause hyperglycemia (a sharp increase in blood sugar levels).

As you've already realized, the big priority is eating complex carbohydrates. The fact that there are also complex carbohydrate priorities, the preferred complex carbohydrates are in their natural form and are not processed such as pasta, bread, etc. Balanced consumption of these complex carbohydrates can be part of the daily diet once it is combined in a balanced way. For example, vegetables that are rich in carbohydrates are an excellent option. Quinoa, in all shapes, has a low glycemic value and is rich in fiber. Seeds and all kinds of beans and lentils are also a good option. Sweet potatoes are also considered a high quality carbohydrate.

The steps to keep your insulin level low in your blood over time

1. Avoid as much processed food as possible
2. Avoid sweets and snacks
3. All types of sugar are problematic (fruit consumption is allowed and even recommended)
4. If it comes packed, it is probably not good, and it is best to avoid them (they have added sugars and other substances)

What are the alternatives?

You cannot completely avoid sugar, and you cannot completely prevent your children from eating sugar, but what you can do is to get them used to healthier desserts like fresh fruit, chocolate that is over 70 percent cocoa, a wide variety of nuts, and many more can be a great option as a dessert.

Be sure to reduce as much pre-packaged foods as possible. These foods are full of salts and sweeteners that damage the sense of taste and cause you to forget the true and authentic tastes, and thus reduce your desire to eat fresh foods.

The secret to weight loss

Vegetables, vegetables, vegetables ...

Vegetables can help you or your children to lose weight. When you eat more vegetables during the day, you have less of a desire to eat other things such as sweets. Vegetables are satisfying; high in nutritional values; rich in vitamins, minerals, and fibers; and they satisfy the feeling of satiety.

It is important to understand that vegetables will help weight loss, as long as the vegetables replace other things like sugars, breads, pastas, etc.

The thirty-day vegetable challenge

One of the most effective ways I have come to know to create habits of eating a lot of vegetables that suits both children and adults is the vegetable challenge.

The vegetable challenge is a very enjoyable way for the whole family to help each and every family member to eat more vegetables. What is good is that when you eat more vegetables and eat less of the other unhealthy foods, it will lead to weight loss. Today, because there is a target for a certain amount of pre-determined vegetables, after meeting the same daily task throughout the week, the next week adds another vegetable.

This means that if you eat four vegetables during the first week, the second week starts with eating five vegetables every day. If you cannot accomplish the task during the week and miss the amount of vegetables that you set for the week, you have to do another week of the same amount. A family does not accumulate points during this week and prevents further progress in stages. This means that children and all members of the family can increase the amount of vegetables they eat every day without feeling that they are being asked to, as in a game or small competition between the family members.

You will find the table below in the booklet attached to this book. Write in the name of each member of the family. Whoever has been on the mission for seven days will receive a star (*). One goal is to see who can eat the most vegetables by the end of the week (and they will receive two stars (**).

Family	Sun.	Mon.	Tue.	Wed.	Thu.	Fri.	Sat.	Total	Stars
Daddy	3	4	3	3	4	3	4	24	*
Mommy	3	3	2	2	4	2	4	19	-
Jon	3	3	3	1	4	3	5	22	-
Jessica	3	4	3	5	4	3	4	26	**
Roxanne	3	3	4	3	4	3	3	23	*

In the workbook, you can get the full thirty-day table for the full vegetable challenge.

If you need to download the workbook, the download link is at the beginning of the book.

Tips for the success of the vegetable challenge

- Every meal has vegetables, so every time you eat, you accumulate a good number of vegetables. At first, there will be no problem meeting the goals, but the larger the goal grows, the more challenging it will be to start from a higher number if you are not used to eating vegetables.
- The vegetables should be available and accessible to the children. The vegetables should be fresh and ready to eat. Prepare a plate of fresh vegetables every day, and place it in the refrigerator. If you cut or peel some vegetables, you can add lemon to keep them fresh.

A house with an overweight child

First of all, we talked about how parents are role models.

All the rules that apply to the child include the parents!

The child will eat what the parent prepares, meaning, if he has healthy food, he will eat it. If there is less healthy food on the plate, he will eat it. The child depends on the parent and what they put on his plate. The role of the parents is that there will always be a variety of available food that is healthy, and the role of the child is to choose from this variety.

In most cases, children are more easily seduced by temptations and prefer to choose the less healthy options that are usually more tasty. If we take a child and put him in front of a large tray of sweets and chocolates, cakes and cookies, and a second tray of vegetables and fruit, what he will choose is pretty clear. He will probably choose the tray of sweet food. If I gave this choice to an adult, they would make the same choice as the child and go to the candy tray. If the child does not choose the sweet option and chooses the vegetables instead, this is probably a sign that the parents did a really good job.

How much weight should a child lose if he or she is overweight?
It is not always necessary for a child to lose weight. In many cases, children under the age of 7 are recommended to maintain their weight, because at these ages, the children are not tall enough. If necessary, it is very important that the decline be controlled and gradual.

There is no need for extremism. Daily physical activity and balanced eating will do the job in a much more effective way, and the results will remain over time.

The process is gradual and is not perceived as something extreme that can be experienced as a trauma. The child should lose weight. A correct decline is a slow and gradual decline—between 1 to 4.5 pounds per month. Of course, it also depends on the child's initial weight and health. In order to know a little more accurately how much the child needs to lose, you can use the BMI table that appears in the book and in the attached workbook.

If you need to download the workbook, the download link is at the beginning of the book.

In addition, it is always advisable to seek professional advice, which will help to build a gradual work plan for the child's weight loss.

Should we hide the candy, yes or no?

One of the common mistakes is the hiding of snacks and sweets from the child with the intention that the child will not eat them. Hiding sweets from the child may create many bad situations. The first time they find a sweet, it will feel like a treasure hunt. When you hide treats from the child, it is an action that may cause the child to be obsessed with food the moment he realizes that the food is at home, but it is hidden.

He will seek the treats and get excited, because he is not supposed to find them. And, once he finds the food, his eating will be emotional and disproportionate, and he will have no self-control. So, it is very important that you avoid these experiences. All the foods that you know are unhealthy (chocolates, candy, cookies, etc.) should not even enter your house. The moment it does enter the house, it will be like a matter of seduction for your children.

It is very important to involve the child in the process of removing sweets from the home. The child knows what is going on, and he will notice if things suddenly change at home. Explain to him that you have decided that the whole house will start a healthier lifestyle, and everyone will do it together. Take note of the change that you are making, get them to do the same process, and the children's adjustments will be much easier. You are invited to return to the chapter where we talked about setting goals as a family. This part will help you make the transition easier and more efficient.

Avoidance of foods

As I mentioned earlier, if there are foods that are less healthy and tastier, the child will probably choose them over vegetables. So, how do you solve the problem and make the child simply not eat the bad foods? The truth is that the way is very simple, if the child eats at home!

If you do not bring certain foods home, then you simply will not have to deal with what is allowed and what is forbidden, because it just is not within reach. One of the things that most parents do not want to do at home is to create a different attitude and different behavior between each of the children at home. The parents want everyone to feel the same and that no one will be deprived.

Do not blame the child for eating a lot of sweets. It's not her fault, that's what she likes and that's what she's used to. We all have a tendency toward sweet food and junk food. But, in the end, you are the ones who do the shopping and the children eat what is available at home. Most of the time, children eat at home or bring food from home. If you take out those foods that are considered "problematic" from the environment accessible to the child, then you simply will not have the option to eat the same things. And, if the child is hungry, he will choose one of the available and healthy foods at his disposal.

In the event that the child eats at school or in a post-school setting like lunch, check the food they serve. There are times when the food served there is no better than junk food. Check what your children are given to eat and, if necessary, bring the food to your children.

Avoiding food and sweets as a reward or punishment

Do not treat food as a reward or a punishment. It is not recommended to use food to change a child's behavior. It is very common today when a sad child, or an angry child, or any other state of negative emotion, is upset to give him a candy to cheer him up. And, from the other side, as soon as a child does something good or behaves okay he will make it a candy prize.

This way of rewarding the child is very problematic and can have consequences. Habits that are developed in the child will have an effect in the future as an adult. Over the years, the same habits become more and more established, and the longer the habit has gone on, the harder it will be to make a change.

What is conditioning?
Conditioning is a concept that comes from the world of psychology. Conditioning can create an activation of emotions and a certain behavior in connection with a particular action. For example, every time a child does something good or wants to be comforted, he will turn to that comforting candy or food, because that is what they were given each time they were sad to make them happy. It is important to avoid making connections between food and actions.

One of the most well-known experiments in history on this subject is Ivan Pavlov's experiment.

So, what was the experiment?

Pavlov conducted an experiment to investigate a phenomenon: he gave a number of dogs food and, at the same time, rang the bell. He performed the experiment several times. The first time he rang the bell, the dogs came and they were without drool. The second time he rang the bell and gave them food. He repeated the same action again and again, and he noticed that, after several times, when he rang the bell and the dogs arrived, the dogs arrived with drool in their mouths, even though they had not received the food. The experiment went on and on. Eventually, all he had to do was ring the bell and the dogs would start drooling without even seeing the plate of food. What Pavlov did was create a connection between the action (ringing the bell) to a physical condition (the dogs drool).

This experiment can show the power of every action taken in parallel to another action, and the connection it creates between those situations.

Should we not eat sweets, ever?

First of all, let's start from the fact that it is permissible and even recommended to enjoy all these delicious foods from time to time. But, what is important is that it is not accessible all the time and every day. Insulin resistance is produced from long-term exposure.

For example, if you have a meal at home and your guests bring desserts, make sure that at the end of the meal you bring what is leftover to your guests, so they can take it home.

Do not leave food in the refrigerator that should be avoided.

Quite simply, if the bad food is not around, there is nothing to avoid. You may think you cannot keep an eye on your child all day long and see everything he does. You can't control what he puts in his mouth all day long with friends and at school. But, the thing is, you don't have to!

First of all, it is reasonable to assume that eighty percent of what your child eats is at your house. So, there is nothing to worry about. A treat every now and then is okay. He should not feel that he is not allowed ever. It's a matter of time before he slowly learns what is better for him and what is healthier and why he should eat certain foods. This means that your child will learn to make better decisions on his own. But for the whole process to be effective and usable, there is no need to make it difficult for the child, so just don't keep those foods in the house.

It's a matter of attitude

One of the things you do not want to do is take a child and make the transition from a healthy diet to a tragedy. It's all about attitude, and the way you show it to a child. If you see enthusiasm for healthy food, the chances are much higher that he will cooperate with you. If you say things like, "Today we will have to give up pizza and eat salad and eggs instead," it will be accepted differently. Do not show the transition as something that has to be abandoned. Make the transition gradual and in cooperation with the child. If it becomes a tragedy for him, he will not cooperate with you.

Education for proper nutrition

Proper nutrition and habits go together. Proper nutrition education contains a wide range of educational values such as listening, self-love, responsibility, rejection of gratification, balance, and even boundaries!

Education for proper nutrition is, of course, in the hands of the parents or the authoritative figure who raises the child. It seems that, in recent years, it has become increasingly difficult to educate for proper and healthy nutrition because of a number of key factors. If both parents are building a career in parallel with raising the children, it is difficult to find the time to prepare healthy food at home. So, parents start using more readily available foods, such as frozen or prepared foods. In addition to this, there are many more temptations, snacks, sweets, and advertisements that support and entice children and adults to want more and more of the same things.

What is the best way to teach proper nutrition?
The best way to teach is not to teach; there is no better way to do it than to be a role model. Children are the best imitators, and what they see the parents do, they will do themselves, without the need for explanations or preaching. Once a child sees his parent doing a certain thing, he will think it is something that is right to do, because his parent does it.

Teaching proper nutrition

Food groups

- Teach your children to understand what they are eating.
- What is the importance of these foods?
- Why is it important to eat them?
- What do they contribute to?
- What are the food groups and the differences between them—proteins, fats, and carbohydrates? Teach them which foods belong to the same group. For example, is white bread considered as carbohydrates, fats, or proteins? This knowledge is very basic and can greatly contribute to children who can understand on their own what is better for them to eat so they can make the decisions on their own.
- Explain to them what vitamins and essential nutrients are in every food through stories, reading, or invented stories on the subject. What is nice is that the storytelling isn't just for bedtime. It can be at any time, and it can be incorporated during the cooking and shopping processes.

- Teach them while doing joint work. When did you last make dinner together?
- Teamwork - organize the whole family and prepare a healthy meal together so that the learning will be experiential, while teaching the children what foods are considered healthier, why they help, and why is it preferable to something else?
- Take the kids with you to the supermarket, so they can see what you choose. Here you can have fun and give tasks to the children during the shopping trip to activate their creativity and make it a learning experience, and not just a task that must be done.
- Share with your children and make them an active part of your choices. Teach them why you are making the choices you make.

Let children take an active part in shopping, cooking, and other activities related to these topics. Children learn best by watching the way parents work. Share your choices and decisions with them. All this will help to produce an interest around the food in different ways. Cook with the child. Let him touch different textures and different foods with his hands. Let her smell spices. Ask him to come up with creative ideas for food that can be prepared next time. Decide that every week you will give them something new to taste, and treat it like a game. Let the child take an active part in bringing the food to the plate, and understand what the food is going through before it reaches the plate. You don't want them to think of food as something that comes out of the oven.

- Teach your children what balance is.
- What is a healthy lifestyle? There is no need to use words like diet or weight control, which can be perceived as something wrong with the child and a change must be made. You can use the word balanced eating or a healthy lifestyle.
- Teaching a child about a healthy and balanced diet will help them make better decisions about nutrition.

Give responsibility to the child

Explain to the child according to their age and level of understanding, that it is in her hands and that she is responsible for her body, because she has only one body. You will do everything you can, and you will not fill the house with sweets and say that it is their responsibility. Give them all the means and all the health options you can offer them, and they will choose from these options.

Teach your children about their bodies and foods. Give them the tools to make the right decisions on their own.

Teach them to take responsibility and take an active part in nutrition-related issues at home, whether it's helping to prepare a meal or shopping. Give them the feeling that they are an active part of what happens on the subject.

Sweets every day

As soon as a child is accustomed to eating dessert after a meal, or a daily dessert, it can cause the child to have a regular habit of eating sweet foods. If he does not really have the desire or need for something sweet, it can still become a habit that leads him to consume something sweet. The problem begins to form when the child did not even think about it or did not want anything sweet but the parent nevertheless brought him a sweet snack or candy. If he did not ask, then there is really no need to offer sweets to him. He will not miss anything if he does not eat the candy. There is no problem eating candy from time to time, but there is no need to suggest it to him. In the event that the child is used to desserts, try to replace those sweets with healthy desserts such as fruits and nuts.

If the child is already used to eating dessert at the end of a meal, you have to start creating the feeling that he will get the candy, but at another time (you are invited to go to the deferral section). It gently postpones gratification each time a little more. This is a process in which you have to make it clear to the child that it's okay that he loves sweets, and he can eat them, but just not now. Avoid telling the child not to ask for candy, and just tell him that tomorrow he can have another candy, maybe two pieces. He needs to break the same habit of eating a candy or dessert at a certain time during the day. As your child grows, it is easier to explain and share your child's decisions about nutrition and how to choose healthy foods.

Listening to the body

Today, more than ever, it is difficult to distinguish between "real" hunger and "imaginary" hunger.

There are several types of hunger. It is important that the parents first distinguish between all the different feelings that each person has on a daily basis. It is sometimes very difficult to distinguish between those feelings that can be interpreted in the same way. Once the parent learns to recognize and differentiate between all these feelings, she can also teach her child to distinguish between those feelings and situations.

Which kinds of hunger exist?

- *Boredom* - sometimes you want food because you're bored, and it's something to do.
- *Thirst*- sometimes a feeling of thirst can be translated incorrectly and that person or child may think he is hungry.
- *Hunger from the eyes* - the person is not really hungry but, because they can see all the temptations and good foods, he can think he is hungry.
- *Emotional* - a situation in which a person uses food as emotional compensation or as a safe haven. The person is not necessarily hungry; they have more of an emotional need for food. In many cases, it is difficult for the person to see the difference in what is interpreted as hunger.
- *Physical* - is the condition when a person is really hungry, and the body requires food, because they haven't eaten for several hours. The brain signals that one should eat, and it is expressed with a sense of hunger.

174

Keeping a diary for the different types of hunger
So, how do you get to know those feelings and how can you tell them apart? First of all, what we do is pay attention to the feeling that is interpreted as hunger and check with ourselves what the body goes through and what it feels like.

Allow answers for the following questions:

• What kind of hunger is this?

• Where does it come from?

At first, it may be difficult to pay attention to the same feeling and where it comes from. One way to improve the identification of these feelings is that for a whole week, before you eat something, write down how you felt before that eating action. Were you sad, happy, or bored? Were you watching TV? Were you at work?

Write down which food you ate and at what time, and you will have more accurate tracking.

The same action will monitor how you act in different situations during the day with food, and you can actually map the same feelings that make you eat, and situations where you eat unnecessarily. Once you identify those situations, you can more easily work to change those habits and replace them with new habits that will help. For example, if you have noticed that you are usually looking for something to eat while watching television, and that eating is for employment, then, instead of eating snacks and sweets, you can replace it with healthier foods. This follow-up will help you see where it's harder for you and which situations put you in more stress or any other emotional state that makes you eat.

This exercise makes you think for a second before doing the action. The very fact that you stop for a second and check what happens to yourself at the moment is actually the exercise itself. Managing a diary can be very helpful at first to take this time out and concentrate on exactly what you are going through at the moment.

You can find the nutrition diary in the workbook.

the download link is at the beginning of the book.

Family meals

It is not easy to organize a family meal. It requires preparation and organization, especially for those who want to do the meals several times a week. But, with a little effort, you can do it with proper planning. Various studies have shown that children who eat meals with their parents suffer less from obesity because eating together neatly around the family table makes it very easy to consume healthy food. It is much more likely that we will eat more vegetables as part of a family meal.

According to a study published in the February 2015 issue of the *Journal of Pediatrics*, there is a link between family meals during adolescence and a lower chance of obesity at an older age. In the study, researchers from the University of Minnesota and Columbia University followed approximately 2,000 adolescents for ten years. They found that the higher the frequency of family meals during adolescence, the lower the incidence of obesity. The researchers conclude that family meals have a protective effect against future obesity and recommend at least one or two family meals during the week.

Benefits of a family meal
- In a family meal, parents are a personal example. This is an opportunity to convey healthy verbal and nonverbal messages: the fact that children see their parents eating different foods encourages them to experience them.
- Beyond the fact that it has all the health effects of a family meal, it also has a great impact on the daily

life of the child and those children who eat family meals on a regular basis.

- Better grades - A similar survey conducted by the Columbia University's Addiction Prevention Center found that adolescents who ate family meals five or six times a week were 30% more likely to have high scores than adolescents who ate less often with their parents.
- Less Stress - In addition to this, a family meal also has an effect on stress. Teenagers who eat with the family at a frequency of five to seven times a week suffer about 40% less stress in their lives. The reason for this is that the conversation, the sharing, and the involvement of the parents reduce the feeling of stress significantly.
- Eating disorders - Because of the good relationship between family members created around family time and the support and healthy habits that such a meal promotes, the risk of developing eating disorders is lower. In a study of 2,400 teenaged girls aged 9 to 19 in the United States over a decade, girls who ate family meals more often had fewer eating disorders and related behaviors.
- Less addictions - Parental involvement in children's lives is critical to prevent addictions and other habits that can hurt them. One of the simplest ways for parents to notice the same situations and be there for their children on time is simply to sit together for family dinners.

All these benefits are simply amazing and there are many other advantages that are not mentioned here about the impact and importance of family meals. It is amazing how such a small thing can create such a great and significant change in the lives of parents and children.

Tips for regular family meals

- First of all, decide that it is important enough for you. Once you give it a high place in your priorities, it will be much easier to find time for it. Make it a family goal.
- Build it gradually. If you are not having family meals at all, you don't have to jump straight to seven family meals a week. Start a family meal at the end of the week and another one in the middle of the week and, over time, increase the frequency. It is important to note that family meals are usually more convenient to do in the evening when the entire family is usually at home. If you are more comfortable with other times, then arrange it accordingly.
- Not every meal must be a project of cooking and preparation. Even relatively light meals of eggs and vegetables will do the job.
- Turn off the TV screens while sitting at the table, and no smartphones. The message to children is that this is a time devoted exclusively to the family.
- If there is a difficulty in finding the time for the family meal, you can talk to the children and try to determine with them how much time they will have for the meal. If there is a TV show they like, try to consider it.

Boredom and weight gain

Combining a lack of physical activity with eating high-carbohydrate and sugary foods causes obesity in children. Eating out of boredom is very common among obese children. Today, career parents are at work late, and the children are often at home alone playing on Xbox or on the Internet. Today it is less common for kids to go down to play on the street with friends. If the children do meet with friends, many times it comes down to meeting at someone's house where they all play Xbox.

Fatigue and boredom are both outcomes of a "negative" emotional state that leads people to overeat and gain weight. Many times, the word "I'm hungry" can be replaced by the words "I'm bored." You can see this phenomenon when the child has finished a plate full of food and then has no occupation. So, after a short time, he says he's hungry, although there is no chance he will be hungry after such a meal.

Have you ever had such a busy day that you simply got sucked into it until you finally said to yourself, "Wow! It's been a whole day, and I haven't eaten yet?" Or, on the contrary, do you know those days when you're at home or at work and you're so bored, and you are just waiting for the day to end, and find yourself looking for something else to eat over and over again?

What should be done when children eat when they are bored?
If you are at home, one of the most common and simple ways to distract a child until the next meal time is playing with them or giving them activities that will relieve them of the boredom. The problem is that it can be very exhausting every day to entertain children and, of course, it is not always possible.

The goal is to make children more active and healthier. You will need to think about other ways to spend time in activities other than watching TV. So, what you can do is to fill the child's day with activities such as classes, meeting friends, cycling, etc. Once the child is busy, he will not even think about food because he has employment. Remember, children are an energy bomb—they owe and demand the release of this energy. If there is no way to discharge this energy, then the child will have to unload it elsewhere—for example, food!

Tips - for proper and balanced eating

Eating in front of the TV can affect you in several ways

- You do not pay attention to what you eat or how much you eat when there is a TV in the background.
- Employ the jaw and pay no attention to food entering the mouth.
- The sense of satiety is not always directly felt because of the dishonest attention to eating, which leads to a greater consumption of food.

One way to deal with the uncontrolled eating of food is simply not to eat in front of the screen. Give the meal the right place at the dining table. As soon as the TV is turned off, the food will be more controlled and given the attention needed. Your children will fill much faster, because they are attentive to their body.

Big eyes

Use small dishes at meals. Studies have shown that people eat more if their food is on a large plate.

One experiment showed that children poured twice as much cereal into a larger bowl. And another experiment found that people pour 37% more liquid into wide, shorter glasses than tall thin glasses with the same volume. It is therefore important to pay attention, not only to the food served, but also for the way it is served.

Take the time
Teach your children to stop everything and concentrate on the meal. Teach them to enjoy the meal and to enjoy eating. Teach them to eat slowly and to listen to their bodies. Eating slowly in a calm state helps you to notice more quickly the sense of satiety and prevents you from eating more food.

Picky food eaters

Has your child gotten stuck on three foods? Would he not try anything else? This can indicate that he is picky or even very picky. There are situations in which children develop selectivity over the years; whereas, as little children, they would eat everything. Many of those same children choose to play a game of strength against their parents. Once the parent "surrenders" to the manipulations of the child, the same selectivity can stay with him until a late age, and sometimes for life. One of the problems of food selectivity is that it can lead to deficiencies. Because the variety of food is small, the nutritional values that the child needs may be missing. It is important to understand that even if foods are healthy, deficiencies can occur.

Many times, in these situations, the parent can find himself preparing the same foods repeatedly that the child likes. "But the main thing is that he eats." But the problem is that once the parent gives him the same foods again and again, the child develops a fixation on the same foods, and that prevents him from experimenting with new foods.

What can you do with a picky kid?
- First of all, patience is required.
- One of the ways to deal with over-selectivity is to continue to prepare some of the foods the child enjoys eating, but also add new foods that the child has avoided or has not yet eaten.
- Graduation can help the child because the child will not feel frustrated that he has nothing to eat, and, on the other hand, an option is opened for

him to recognize new foods that do not replace the foods he likes.

- Keep in mind that children need to get used to the taste of the food, the smell, and even the color.
- If your child will not taste a dish the first time you introduce it to your child, you should not give up. At the next meal, the child may agree that the dish will sit on his plate. At a meal after that, he may still not agree to eat it. It can go on like this again and again until, suddenly, after the fifth time, he is willing to try it.
- Give him time to get used to the food. He does not know the taste or the texture, and there is nothing to get excited about. It can take a little longer. You can always try the same dish, and then try it again after a few days. A child may love a certain food only after a few meals in which he has had the opportunity to know it.

Remember- It is important not to struggle and not to force the child to eat. Once there is a struggle between the parents and a child around the subject of food, the child will sometimes want to show his power and position and just will not eat to show his strength. Ultimately, the child is the one who decides what goes into his body and what doesn't. If the child does not want to eat, it is not necessary to force him or tell him that if he does not eat he will remain hungry, or that there are children who have nothing to eat. There is no need to use manipulations to make the child eat. You do not have to run after him with the food so he can eat, or continue to press and convince him to eat, even if the child does not eat anything. Patiently tell him, "You are probably not hungry now, you can eat later."

It is very important to never give him a snack or candy when he has not eaten his meal.

Experiences with new foods

Play with the food

It is permissible to play with food and even preferred. There are many children who do not like to eat anything, but taste is something that can be purchased. The eating experience should be enjoyable and the food itself should be enjoyable.

How do you make food fun? One way is to bring an omelet and vegetables to the table and then arrange it in the form of a smiling face.

You can use this way to introduce new foods to your child that she would not eat until today. As long as you are interested in the food and make it a little different, sometimes it is enough to make the child eat and experiment with new foods, because it's not just food; it's also a game. Think of ideas together with the child, and let her mess with the food in her hands and get to know the foods closely. This can help her to connect to those foods she was not used to eating.

Tips

When dealing with a picky child, it is very important to direct the focus on the good things the child did. "Well done, finishing the cucumber." Instead of saying, "Why didn't you eat the tomato?"

- Communicate with the child and ask him which food he likes more.
- It is important to rule out medical problems. First of all, it is recommended that you see your doctor to discover any physical problems, such as swallowing problems, heartburn, digestive problems, hypersensitivity to certain textures, etc.

Water

Water is the drink the body needs most, as water is important for maintaining good health. The body constantly loses water through perspiration, breathing, and urine. In order to maintain our bodies, we need a constant fluid supply throughout the day.

Water is the main component of our bodies. The child's body contains about 75% water, and the brain contains about 85% water. Water plays an important role in all bodily functions.

- Regulates body temperature
- Aids the digestive system
- The water in our blood leads nutrients and oxygen to all parts of our bodies
- Greases joints
- Protects organs
- Removes waste
- Participates in growth processes

Drinking water habits in children

Parents are a personal example and they affect their children in the best possible way. Children who grow up in a house where sweet drinks are part of the daily routine will have difficulty getting used to drinking water. Targeting the child to drink water is an excellent basis for a healthy life. It is important to give children a personal example, so be careful to drink plenty of water at home. Most children do not drink the recommended amount of water, which is one of the reasons children are at greater risk of dehydration. Children also produce more heat than adults and adapt to heat more slowly.

Children are not aware of the signs of dehydration and do not drink enough water. When the child feels thirsty, he has already lost 2% of his body fluids. Such dehydration can lead to difficulty concentrating, headaches, and even a decline in cognitive and physical performance. Lack of water is the main cause of fatigue during the day. Therefore, it is important to drink water not only when we are thirsty.

Drinking water and losing weight

As we have already said, most of our bodies are made of water. Once the body is saturated with water, it can function more efficiently. Water helps the digestive system and other systems function more efficiently. The same efficiency helps the body to do the same processes properly and, as a result, it can help weight loss.

Many people can misinterpret hunger as thirst, and when a person drinks enough water during the day, he will feel fuller and will have less desire to eat unnecessarily. It is important to drink water half an hour before the meal and at the end of the meal. Drinking water causes a faster feeling of satiety if you drink it half an hour before the meal. The recommendation is two cups of water (500 mL). This will help you to eat more moderately and help you to make better decisions in the selection of food and quantities.

Sweet drinks

Sweet drinks are not nutritious. The drinks are made of sugars or sugar substitutes and are filled with food coloring, flavors, smells, and other substances. The drinks are harmful in terms of empty calories—in small children, it may replace a real meal. Drinking sweet drinks proved to be one of the significant factors in obesity in children. A reduction in drinking sweet drinks and developing a habit of drinking water have been shown in studies to prevent obesity in children, and as significant contributors to slimming overweight children. In view of the increase in obesity among children, they should be more careful to drink water. It is a simple habit to acquire, and its efficiency is proven. For parents whose children are drinking only juices, it is advisable to gradually lower the concentration of the juice every day until the children get used to the water.

Tips for drinking more water

- When leaving the house, equip your children with a bottle.
- Make sure the water is accessible to your children. A water bar or bottled mineral water should be placed in a visible and easy-to-reach location.
- Reduce the purchase of the sweetened and sugared drinks at home and replace them with water.
- Drink water before and during exercise.
- Children love explanations - explain and teach your child how important the water is to our body's health.
- Parents are the best personal example for the children, so, drink plenty of water and your children will learn from you!

- Encourage them to drink water. Ice can be added in different forms to the water, which will turn the drinking into fun. You can use special glasses or special bottles, and they should be chosen by the children.
- A bottle is an excellent way to measure how much the child drank in the bottle and allows the child to follow how much he drank.
- To harness the children to the task, it is possible to decide that by noon a bottle should be finished, and this will mobilize them for action.
- You can decorate the bottle, create intimacy, and connect the child to the bottle (all depending on their age, of course).
- Water can be varied in different ways by extracting herbal teas with cold water, so that water is obtained with color and taste without adding sugars.

Recommendations for drinking water

How do you know that your child drinks enough water?

- *Color* is the best measure. During the day, the urine should be transparent. If there is little yellowish or dark urine, it indicates that there is little fluid in the body. This does not apply to the morning urine, because you do not drink water all night long.
- *Smell* of urine is more acute when there is not enough liquid in the body. When you drink enough water, the urine color becomes clear and the smell disappears.
- *The number of times* a child needs to visit the toilet ranges between three to nine times a day. This indication should be taken with limited care, since those who do not drink enough will not go to the toilet often enough.

190

So, how do you know how much water your children need to drink in a day? You can go over the table below and see the recommended data for daily water consumption in children.

Liters	Age
0.7	0.5-0
0.8	1-0.5
1.3	3-1
1.7	8-4
2.4	13-9Boys
2.1	13-9Girls
3.3	18-14Boys
2.3	18-14Girls

Chapter 5:
Physical activity

The importance of physical activity

The importance of exercise is spoken in almost every way, whether it is through the Ministry of Health, on television, or in schools. Physical activity has a huge impact on the health, especially on those who suffer from obesity or morbid obesity. Physical activity has a great influence beyond weight loss on the state of physical health and mental health and takes a significant part in all matters related to the raising of self-image, body image, and self-confidence.

Metabolic syndrome and physical activity
The metabolic syndrome describes a set of risk factors:
- Heart disease
- Obesity, morbid obesity
- Hypertension
- An increase in triglycerides and a decrease in HDL cholesterol (the "good" cholesterol)
- Insulin resistance (a pre-diabetic condition in which insulin efficiency is poor and therefore the pancreas secretes a greater amount of insulin to prevent the rise in blood sugar)
- Et cetera

Exercise in a sitting world
Disturbing data from Western countries demonstrate that about a quarter of children do less than twenty minutes of intensive physical activity per week, which is far less than the usual recommendations. The problem is more common in adolescence when adolescents spend more and more time on phone and social networks.

But, the same lack of activity in youth is mostly due to a lack of activity in early childhood and a lack of healthy exercise habits. Today, preschool-aged children perform less physical activity than before; they spend time on phones and computers. Despite everything, we know about the many benefits exercise has to offer, yet people are less active than ever. Studies show that 31% of the world's population does not exercise adequately. This is true both for developed countries and for developing countries, and for both adults and children. Some health experts refer to this state of inactivity as "new smoking" because of the considerable health damage it causes, which is no less than smoking, like the metabolic syndrome we talked about earlier.

Today compared to the past

In the past, humans were much more physically active, and they made long journeys from one side of a continent to the other side. They would work very hard physically for the food they had at home, and they would build and assemble everything with their own hands because there was no other way. Men had to be strong to survive. They would build houses, carriages, and war equipment with their own hands. Women cooked, and carried buckets full of water and bags of food with amazing weights on their shoulders. You can see all of this even in our third-world countries today. Women carried weights and performed many actions that required great strength that would not shame any bodybuilder in the gym.

Today, what seems legitimate and so simple, like drinking water, used to be a lot of effort in the past. Today, we walk two meters, open the faucet, and we have plenty of water. Humankind is indeed the most developed creature on earth. We have learned how to use the resources available, so we can work less hard.

But what happens today is that people do not need to be physically active to function and live, so our daily conduct requires almost zero percent effort. We drive a car to work, sit in an office for hours, and then go back to the house and watch TV. Basically, you can do anything without being active at all. There are many people who avoid gyms or exercise because they say it's not for them. But as you've already realized, there's no such thing! The human body is meant to be active, period. The many gyms and physical activities allow you to do what your body should be doing every day.

The body builds itself according to its activity

The body is built according to what it does. In the past, if a person was physically active and had to lift and drag and build things, his body was built in such a way that he could withstand the same loads. The body would build more muscle mass to stand under the same weights, and their bone density would be higher due to the same weight resistance. Today, on the other hand, there is no such resistance, and our bodies are mostly inactive. What happens to a body that is inactive?

This situation can be likened to a Ferrari. Instead of filling the engine with fuel, taking care of the car regularly, and traveling with it on the roads, what happens if you just take the Ferrari and put it under the sun without moving it

196

at all. Over time, the Ferrari will crumble into dust. It doesn't matter how beautiful the car was or that each part was hand-made. Eventually, the frame will be destroyed by rust, no matter how much money they originally invested in it. The thing is, a car is designed to move; a vehicle that does not move and sits in place for many years will simply be destroyed!

On the other hand, a vehicle that has been properly treated and traveled can continue to travel for decades and be in excellent condition. This is also true of the human body. Every day the person is not active, the body accumulates "rust" and degenerates and becomes weaker and more fragile.

What happens when you want to pick up a piece of paper from the floor?

Oops ... herniated disk, weak muscles, weak skeleton, and there is a lack of flexibility. This leads to the simplest activity leading to an injury. Lack of physical activity increases the chances of being significantly more vulnerable to injuries.

Children's favorite activity
Today, children prefer to spend their time in front of their screens, rather than go outside to play. Many times, parents do not know how to deal with this, and they do not know how to set boundaries, which leads to the children finding themselves sitting in front of the television screens and the smartphones.

Today's technology enables parents to find activities for the child in seconds, whether it is computer games, smartphones, etc. The problem is the dosage and the place it takes in the daily life of each child.

Everything must be in its own place and its own time. The same way it is not healthy to eat only chocolate or fast food, it is not healthy to sit in front of the TV for hours without performing any activity.

A few years ago, kids would meet up with friends after school and play football for hours or ride a bicycle. People used to be much more active but, because of the development of technology, there is an ever-increasing possibility that children will spend time inside the house without moving from the sofa. It is very important to construct a balance in children between TV viewing and exercise.

The effect of physical activity on the physical aspect

Physical activity has a great impact on the physical condition. We will review some of the benefits and effects of physical activity on the body. Physical activity helps to strengthen the immune system and reduces the chances of suffering from many chronic diseases and various physical problems such as heart disease, vascular disease (such as stroke), high blood pressure, osteoporosis, elevated cholesterol levels, and more.

A significant percentage of children and adolescents who are obese and morbidly obese suffer from insulin resistance due to obesity. This condition can develop later into diabetes if it is not treated in time. This type of diabetes, which was previously common in adults only, is becoming increasingly common in children and adolescents in Western countries where physical activity decreases from year to year.

An increase in the prevalence of obesity in children has led to a marked increase in the incidence of diseases that were not common in children in the past and could only be seen in older adults. Physical fitness can minimize the damage and complications of obesity. Studies among adults have taught us that a fat person in good shape is significantly protected from mortality and obesity complications. In fact, poor physical fitness in adults is a significant risk factor for mortality, even more than smoking or various chronic diseases such as diabetes. This means that even a person of high weight can benefit from the good effects that exercise has to offer. In addition, it was found that exercise can prevent different types of cancer.

Physical activity in the mental and emotional aspect
Physical activity has a major impact on our mental state. It is now known that one of the biggest causes of diseases is stress and anxiety, and the same conditions can develop to a chronic level. Today, more and more people suffer from diseases that were not common in the past. Chronic stress has a very big effect on the body and can cause many physical problems like heart disease, type 1 and 2 diabetes, and it can even lead to depression. A meta-analysis published in 2008 examined 49 studies of physical activity and the effect on people's mental states, and it showed a significant reduction in mental stress of those who

exercised regularly, compared to control groups that did not exercise.

Exercise also had an advantage in relation to anxiety therapy. It's amazing how much exercise can affect your mental state. The simplest and most accessible thing can make a significant difference in the lives of so many people. It's a pity that medicine does not appreciate it enough and does not give precise instructions for exercising to cope with anxiety and depression, in addition to the usual treatment.

Physical activity should be part of the treatment process for any person suffering from depression or anxiety. Another study examined three meta-analyses of the effect of exercise on different types of mental stress, and exercise was a proven way to reduce mental stress.

Regular participation in physical activity can help children mentally in many ways

- Lowers general voltage levels significantly
- Improves mood
- Improves self-confidence
- Increases self-image and body image
- Improves academic performance
- Improve memory and concentration
- Improves thinking processes
- Improves concentration
- Improves decision-making
- Helps everyone to have a better sleep; lack of sleep has a direct connection to chronic stress; a lack of sleep can greatly impair daily functioning, and it also affects our mental state

- Et cetera

When will we see the results of regular activity?
The benefits of physical training begin to accumulate considerably once the exercise becomes permanent and is performed daily over time.

What happens is that the body adjusts to the new demands that are placed on it. This means that the body needs to be exposed to a higher level of difficulty, and once that happens, the body must spend more effort.

A gap is created between what the body was used to doing (without exercise) and what effort it takes when the person starts exercising. Once it happens, the body needs to "catch up" and close the gap created.

What happens while the body catches up?
The lungs lose more oxygen, and, as soon as the breathing becomes deeper and faster, it affects the function of the heart, which pumps more oxygen with each beat.

All of these changes make a person feel more energetic, full of life, and they have improved athletic abilities as a result of improved cardiovascular endurance. Adjustments usually begin within a few weeks after starting to exercise regularly.

These biological changes make a significant change to a person's health condition in the short and long term.

Recommendations for physical activity
You know people who say, "I want a dog in the house, but the problem is that the house is small and the dog will not

have anywhere to spend energy," or "If I had a garden, I would get a dog. I don't want him to get bored all day at home." So it is that children are also very energy-intensive, and they demand the discharge of this energy. When the child lies in front of the television screen, the child is not able to discharge the same energy accumulated in him.

There are various recommendations for exercise in children, but it is usually recommended they perform sixty minutes or more of exercise per day. It is important to remember that this is a cumulative time of physical activity that includes active break time in school, sports classes, etc. So, the activity does not have to be one continuous hour. The time can accumulate over the course of a number of activities during the day. Of course, children who are not used to exercising will do so start gradually until they reach sixty minutes of exercise per day.

As you understand exercise, great importance is attached to every person, both children and adults. The difference between an adult and a preschool child is that it is easier for young people to regain their fitness. So, if your child has not been active until now, there is no need to worry. After a few weeks, the child will be able to do much more, whereas, an adult will take a little longer. It's important to remember that a significant improvement can be seen within a few weeks of starting to exercise.

The World Health Organization recommends the following amounts of physical activity by age

- *5–17 years of age:* Take 60 minutes vigorous exercise every day. More exercise provides more health benefits. Perform activities that strengthen the skeleton and bones at least 3 times a week.

- *18–64 years of age:* It is best to have at least 150 minutes of moderate exercise during the week, or at least 75 minutes of vigorous exercise during the week (or a similar combination of vigorous and moderate activity). For additional health benefits, adults are advised to perform 300 minutes of exercise during the week. Perform muscle strengthening activities (strength training) should be performed 2 weeks or more.

- *Over the age of 65:* It is best to have at least 150 minutes of moderate exercise during the week, or at least 75 minutes of vigorous exercise. There is an additional health benefit in having exercise for 300 minutes (5 hours) per week. People with mobility problems should perform activities that will improve their balance and prevent falls three times a week or more. Muscle strengthening activities (strength training) should be done two times a week or more.

The intensity of physical activity varies among people. To enjoy improved heart/lung health, any exercise should last for at least ten minutes.

Group activities

Exercising in groups helps create new relationships and friendships. Interacting with other children helps your child improve their ability to express themselves, giving them the opportunity to be part of something. And, cooperating with other children can help your child develop self-communication and self-expression qualities. Today there is less interpersonal interaction because of technological advances and the way the children prefer to spend their free time in front of the screens.

What if your child doesn't like sports?

There is no such thing as a child who doesn't like any physical activity. Some children do not like certain sports, so let the child try different kinds of sports. There are children who are more suited to group activities, such as soccer, basketball, gymnastics, and long jump. Look at what your child likes and continue looking until you find the sport he or she enjoys and wants to continue. It is important not to despair that you may never find the framework that the child enjoys. A regular framework of exercise will build habits for future physical activity in the child.

Exercise on a daily basis

It's a great personal example if the parents practice what they preach and spend a significant part of their day to a healthy lifestyle. The kids will naturally want to take part. So, do fun activities together or just play with your kids. You can try football, skateboarding, or rollerblades. You can even walk on the walking path near your home. Experiment with your children in different sports, try new things for variety, and find other areas of interest.

To reach the recommended levels of exercise, it is important that the children accumulate as much time as possible in daily activities. Every bit counts. You can start by not driving the kids everywhere. Walk with them or let them walk alone, if they are old enough, but no electric bicycles. Let them do real physical activity. Remember to encourage them and especially encourage a child who is not used to exercising regularly. Remember, if these exercise habits are conditioned at a young age, it will be easier for them in the future to maintain a proper training framework.

Attention deficit hyperactivity disorder (ADHD) and the connection to television and other media
Today, children and teenagers spend hours and hours watching computer games, telephone screens, and television screens that are frenetic. It is known that the brain is flexible and, during your life, it will change and build itself according to the things it is exposed to. What follows is that a child who sits for many hours in front of those screens will need a lot of stimuli to keep him focused. This is probably one of the reasons why so many children today find it difficult to maintain concentration over time, such as reading books and activities that are less frenetic.

Studies are being conducted to determine whether there is a connection between exposure to computer games and the development of attention deficit disorders. Researchers from the United States have conducted extensive cross-sectional research in children and adolescents. For thirteen months, the researchers interviewed and followed 1,323 children on their TV and computer game viewing habits. During this time, they interviewed the children's teachers and parents and filled out questionnaires for ADHD and other learning problems.

The conclusion of the study was that a lot of television viewing and participation in computer games caused an increase in the prevalence of ADHD and learning disorders in children and young adults. The reason is that in the children's television programs, they get used to short stimuli and a lot of action. Every few seconds, the scene changes in order to keep the viewer focused and alert.

Researchers at Microsoft have found that the time when a person can concentrate in a particular action is getting shorter. According to the study, the time at which the concentration can be maintained is about eight seconds— less than the average time a goldfish can concentrate on a particular action.

TV media and obesity

This is indeed a good employment tool for parents who want to find an activity that will give them quiet time from their children for a short period of time.

There are many advantages to today's computers, whether it's a way to teach children a more interesting way, learning languages, etc. But, most of the free time of children does not deal with computer learning and the development of different abilities. Children mainly play and roam the social networks. Computer watching, means they are not performing any physical activity. In addition to that, when children are in front of the screens, it may cause them to eat more.

Researchers found that boys ate a bigger lunch (163 calories) after playing video games, compared to a meal after an hour spent relaxing. The researchers explained that the mental strain involved in working with a computer may mislead the brain to think that the body burned many calories.

Boundaries for screens

Parents need to wake up! Mobile phones, computers, etc. are things that need to be limited to a certain time during the day. Once you have limited the viewing time and the game time, you can fill this time with activities that will contribute to the child's welfare, whether it's outdoor games, bicycling, box games, or after-school activities. You do not want your child to spend his childhood on his computer screen or cell phone.

He may not spend his childhood, as you did, participating in playground games playing football in the field for hours on end, but he will do a lot more than he does right now. Take all the time that has been created, after you've reduced the amount of computer and TV time, and fill it with physical activity for your kids. Before changing this whole process, it is important to involve your children and explain to them why you chose to make this change. You may encounter resistance, but if you do it with fun activities and bring alternatives that are interesting and special for the children, they will not notice at all that they "gave up" on television.

The recommended time to limit screen hours is a cumulative time of up to two hours per day.

Sleep

Sleep is one of the things that the body must have to survive. The body cannot exist without three main components: food, water, and sleep.

Lack of sleep

Although we know that sleep is important, we are not always aware of the consequences of sleep deprivation. People who sleep less than seven hours a night are much more likely to be overweight. In addition, people who sleep less than four hours a night increase their chances of becoming overweight by 73%. Such an extreme sleep restriction will lead to the desire to eat about 900 extra calories a day. Eating this amount of food beyond the normal amount will cause a significant increase in weight, which will lead to a significantly higher caloric intake than what is needed. In addition to the high calorie consumption, there will be a tendency to eat high carbohydrate and sugary foods in the transition to a high-calorie content.

Today, most of the adult population sleeps around seven hours, and about a third of us are satisfied with six hours of sleep and less. One reason is the electric lightbulb and the screens. A review of sixteen studies of 1.5 million people showed that sleeping for less than seven hours a night was associated with an increased risk of death by 12%.

Infinite cycle

Obesity causes more sleep problems, and a lack of sleep causes obesity.

77% of overweight adults complain of sleep problems and a lack of sleep. There is no answer of what comes first, like the story of the egg and the chicken. Another problem arises because the physiological signs of exhaustion, insomnia, and hunger are similar, and they are confusing signs. People tend to eat when they are actually tired, because they mistakenly think that fatigue is a sign of hunger. A lack of sleep leads to lower judgment, and in addition, people are naturally attracted to foods that provide high energy, meaning their caloric value is higher. Most high calorie foods are foods high in sugars and carbohydrates.

There is also a great significance to the sleep sequence and sleep quality. The body will be more drained of energy, and a lack of energy can lead to immune system problems, injuries, or a lack of energy, and it may contribute to the feelings of anger or sadness. Sleep has a great impact on our daily functioning and significantly improves productivity, alertness, concentration, and learning abilities.

Sleep and hormones
As part of the consequences of lack of sleep, there are also hormonal consequences.

Melatonin- One of the hormones secreted during sleep is melatonin (which is, among other things, a cancer inhibitor). To receive an optimal secretion, sleep at night in total darkness. Melatonin secretions are suppressed in the presence of strong light (mainly sunlight). Studies show that artificial lightbulbs and the monitors of computers and telephones cause us to go to sleep later, they cause sleep disorders, and they may cause sleep pathology in some people.

Garlin- is naturally released at night when we sleep. If you do not sleep long enough, your body does not have enough time to heal and repair damage; therefore, your body will try to correct itself during the day after, if possible. Under these conditions, the body is required to excrete garlin during the day, i.e., at a time that is not optimal for it, and it is known that garlin encourages a desire to eat more carbohydrates. Garlin is produced in the stomach and, as mentioned, encourages your appetite, meaning that a greater amount of garlin in the body will make you want to eat more, which explains the increased consumption of calories due to a lack of sleep

Leptin- is a hormone that has become a garlin in its action. Leptin helps to regulate the level and frequency of hunger. Leptin, in fact, signals to the body that it is satisfied and no longer needs food. Leptin has an important role in reducing the urge and physical desire to eat, but it does not affect the emotional impulse to eat sweets and other carbohydrates. When the body is deprived of sleep, it has trouble processing sugar while lowering the level of leptin, which is supposed to suppress appetite, which also explains eating uncontrollably when tired.

How many hours of sleep are recommended for children?

- Children 3 to 5 years old should sleep between 10 and 13 hours
- Children 6 to 13 years old should sleep between 9 and 11 hours
- Children 14 to 17 years old should sleep between 8 and 10 hours

Tips for improving sleep time and quality

Relaxation- sleep can be disturbed by thoughts or occupations that occur before bedtime. The more active and restless a person is, the worse his sleep will be. One way for sleep to be best utilized is to prepare an hour or two before bedtime. Stop watching TV and using computer/phone screens. Under a subdued light, read a book or enjoy any other calm activity. The low light and calm activity will help you to get ready to go to sleep.

Ways that can help put everyone into a sleepy state

- A shower can sometimes be a difficult project and can create arguments and resistance with the child. A child who does not like to take a shower will enter a more alert state, which will keep him away from the feeling of fatigue.
- Eating two hours before planning for sleep can cause gastric activation and can sometimes cause anesthesia problems and deep sleep.
- Disconnect from electronic devices at least an hour before bed. They are one of the main causes of the disorder of continuous and good sleep. The light that is projected from phones and computer screens and television deceives the brain and causes it to think that it is still day and prevents it

from entering a state of calm before sleep. In addition, the transmitted content can cause a lot of alertness or thought. Today there is a function called a blue light filter, and it can be found in almost any mobile device. It reduces the light that makes the brain think it is still daytime. This is another way to reduce the brain's exposure to blue light earlier in the day. It is easier to get into sleep mode with the blue light filter, but this is not an alternative to using electronic devices. It is best to disconnect from those devices and just open a book.

- Nice and relaxing classical music or the music of nature can be listened to at bedtime.
- Put the child to bed at least half an hour before the time you want the child to go to sleep. During this time, you can read a book to the child.
- If you do any of the above things, they will not survive more than a few pages until their eyes close by themselves.

Ways to increase your child's physical activity

- Limit screen time and computer games during the day to two hours a day.
- Do activities that make children active. It does not have to be training. The word training or sports or fitness can sometimes deter the child from using other words such as a trip, a game, etc.
- Talk to your child and find out what he likes to do and what is more fun for him.
- It is very important to offer a variety of activities for your child. On the one hand, she will not be bored, and, on the other hand, this will allow her to recognize a wider range of activities.
- Coordinate your family activity as a physical activity. Take care of how you spend time together as a family and what your hobbies are. The recommendation is to perform an hour of exercise a day if the child is not used to it. Ten minutes as a start will do the job and then you can slowly increase the amount of time.
- Make sure your child is in an organized physical activity that is part of his daily routine.
- Adopt your daily activity with you and your children from as young as possible and grow up as a family that loves and enjoys physical activity.

Physical activity and preparation for the real life

Physical activity has other good effects, such as mobilizing for action and helping to instill self-discipline, striving to achieve goals, and striving for achievement, excellence, commitment, and perseverance. They are very important for preparing the child for the "real life."

Persistence is a feature of those who do not stop what they are trying do. They are determined to continue, diligent, consistent, and have an uncompromising stubbornness in the face of the temptation to stop the effort. Success in any field, from sports and art to business and career, requires perseverance. There are many people who do not persist in their efforts and who do not succeed, and others get opportunities they do not have. In many cases, these are people who do not persevere in the effort and let go when faced with the difficulties that lie ahead.

The principle of persistence in **physics** states that each body tends to remain in the state in which it is located. If it were at rest, it would strive to remain where it was. If in motion, it would strive to maintain its speed (size and direction). To maintain the movement, there is no need for an external influence. In everyday reality, bodies do not maintain their movement, because it is very difficult to avoid external influences. The stronger the child has the qualities of perseverance and self-discipline, the less he will be affected by the situations he encounters during life. People with very low persistence abilities will be affected by their environment, they will change direction or stop, and they will not persist.

How do you help a child to persevere?
Perseverance is a capacity that can be built. Persistence depends on the number of components. The role of the parent is to help the child find the same interest and give him all the tools needed to build the same quality of persistence by mainly supporting the intention and exposing the child to the abilities inherent in them. For a

child to persevere in a particular field, he has to have an interest in the field, and he must want to continue on the same subject. He should enjoy the activity and love it, and he must believe in himself. Time will create a sense of ability and help assimilate his ability to persevere. The ability to persevere is created when the child performs the action over time after school hours in a hobby, which the child voluntarily invests in. It can be in any field, including sports. This habit will help the child build values of perseverance and self-discipline, coping with difficulties and striving for excellence, and many other qualities that will help him later in life.

"The drops of rain make a hole in the stone, not by violence, but by oft falling."-Lucretius

---

Crisis of perseverance

As in any age, even at a young age, there are moments of crisis. The same situations in a child's life can sometimes be difficult and unpleasant, stressful, confusing, and even bring the child into a situation where he will not want to continue the activity he has been doing.

These moments are the most magical moments. You must be asking yourself why.

These moments will help the child shape his personality and his ability to cope with moments of difficulty. A parent who does not know how to support a child in these situations and does not have the necessary tools to help the child through the crisis can cause the child to never learn to persevere. He may give up easily, or, worse, not even try.

How do you deal with this situation?

What do you do if, after a period of time, the child decides that he wants to retire from the activity he has been pursuing?

Let's do this step by step to see how we can deal with the situation:

- First, check with the child. Ask him/her what they want to stop.
- Turn to the person who supervises the activity, before you decide to make decisions and ask her what happened in the last lessons. Does she know?
- The goal is not to judge those who understand the situation better, and act accordingly.
- Has the child encountered any difficulty? Did the child not succeed in something during practice? Did the child quarrel with one of the other children during practice? Maybe the child was offended.
- It is very important that you do not rush to remove the child from the situation.

If, each time he has a bit of difficulty, he decides to leave, it can create a pattern of a lack of perseverance that can lead to difficult situations to deal with in "real life" in the future, and any small difficulty will become a crisis.

And if all this does not help?
If the child continues to demand that he wants to leave the same activity what do you do?

Give the child a time window of when they can leave the activity. If there is an unusual case and you must remove the child from the activity then do it. But, explain to the child that you understand his desire to leave, but he cannot stop right away; he can only leave in the middle of the year, for example.

This will be enough time to take him through that crisis, and it will not be the reason he decided to leave. If, during this period, the child continues to repeat that he does not want to continue the same activity, and you realize that it is probably a place not suited for him, ask the child what activity he wants to do instead. Does he want to continue the same activity in another framework? Or does he want another activity altogether?

Clarify this, decide together, and then explain to him that if he wants to go to another activity, it's no problem. This will be at the end of the period you said before and, in a few weeks/months, he can move to what he wants to do. After having had a trial lesson, and learned that he liked it, this created a situation where you received his request and understood him.

On the other hand, you gave him a little more time in the old framework, and he may have started to enjoy it again and forget that he wanted to leave. It is important to share this with the same teacher or coach who is training the child. The coach may make a small change. For example, the coach may give him a little more attention which will make him more active in the lesson, and that will be enough for the child to continue.

In some cases, the child is not ready to stay, and you must try to help him stay in the same frame. It is important not to rush to this option but, in case there is no choice, together with the child you will find another area that interests him that he wants to start doing. It is important not to leave the child in a situation where has no activity. He can stop the activity he no longer wants to do but only after he has an alternative activity that he can start immediately.

Personal example

Again, we return to the subject of a personal example. Even here, this subject is very important. A parent who sets a personal example for his/her children in sports will find it much easier to harness their children for action.

You cannot expect your children to do something you do not do yourself. It does not have to be five sessions a week and an hour and a half in the gym. It would be nice if you decide that's what you want to do, but three times a week walking in the neighborhood or cycling for half an hour can do the job for starters. Even a short twenty-minute workout at home several times a week, or doing a workout of four to five minutes a day will also do the job.

It really does not matter where you choose to start. Every step taken and every little change you make will be noticed by your child. If you take this little step, I can assure you that your child's life is going to change.

Your children will start to watch you and the change that is happening to you, and you'll be surprised at how quickly they become interested and ask about what you are doing, and can they take part in your training.

I have prepared a number of enjoyable exercises that require only a few minutes.

You can start today without accessories and without special equipment. You can do the training in your home. They are located at the following address:

www.omgoverweight.com/workouts

In cases where you prefer to go for a walk or workout in the gym, try the next thing—get organized for a workout. Make sure everyone at home knows you are going for a workout. Ask one of the children to bring you your shoes. Ask them to fill your bottle of water. Share what training you are going to do and ask for a hug and a kiss. And ask them to tell you good luck. This makes the children a part of your activity without doing anything. But, what happens when you come back after the activity and share with them what you did? They will feel they were part of it, because they helped you fill the water bottle and gave you a hug and a kiss. Tell them how much the hug they gave you and the kiss they gave you helped you to do the workout.

Family activity

Today, it is not as common for family members to have the opportunity to work as a team and enjoy family entertainment. Don't allow this fast-paced life to keep you from doing enjoyable things with the people you love so much.

Active recreation with all members of the family has many advantages. It formulates the family and makes everyone communicate with each other. Beyond the family activities, there is also a health reward. Children enjoy playing sports without realizing that they are doing sports by playing. Walk or hike together with the family. It can be a great time for family activities, and it is also an opportunity for parents to set a personal example for the children.

The activity should be fun, enjoyable, and not forced. It is important to do fun activities, and make sure that the children enjoy themselves and want to do these activities again. Enjoy, get excited, and push your kids with your enthusiasm. And this is how you create another way that your children are active.

How do you like to spend time together?
Have you ever thought where you spend your quality time with your kids? What is everybody's favorite hobby? What do you like doing together?

There are two main ways to make your family time enjoyable:

- *Non-active* - such as watching television or a film at a movie theater. Of course it will be accompanied by a cola and popcorn, or dinner at a restaurant near the house. In the end, the activity does not involve any physical activity and, in most cases, it involves food.
- *Active* - going out for a walk in nature, bowling, hiking, riding a bike, walking in the neighborhood, or any activity that combines physical activity. These activities help strengthen ties between the parent and the child. Communication between the family and the joint activity "forces" all members of the family to join the task.

Today it is easier than ever to spend family time together without leaving home. Turn on the TV and enjoy a variety of movies, or series, or computer games. There is no problem in passing the family time in this way, but all things should be in the right dosage. Every type of activity has a place as part of the family activity, but it is important to note that inactive activity is not your main activity. If you notice that this is the case, choose activities that will make your family be more active during family time.

Successful family activity

Preparing for training or a family activity is a significant part of the success of the activity. The preparations that will be made before the activity and at the end of the activity will help to harness the children and the whole family to the task before you even start.

As the children take a more active part in preparing for that activity, they will be more attracted to the activity. So, what should be done before engaging in a family activity? You can start with these simple things:

- Anyone can fill the water their own bottle.
- Choose sportswear for the activity. Let the child choose what she wants for that workout a few hours before or even the day before.
- You can make a uniform for the whole family to wear together whenever you go to do a family workout.
- You can buy colored sweaters and every time choose which one to wear.
- At the end of the activity, you will choose, together with the children, what you would like to do in the next family activity.
- Ask your kids what they enjoyed more and enjoyed less. Over time, you will get more enthusiasm for coaching, and the children will have the ability to choose to do what they love and enjoy more.

So, let's start by making a change and, instead of going out and eating ice cream, go for a walk or play soccer.

Ideas for family activities

Sports navigation:

is a rising trend that is very suitable for families. This is a joint activity in different areas, combining orientation, physical activity, and knowledge of new sites. There are different types of tracks that you can choose according to the levels of difficulty, from small children to specialists. The family goes out to find several stations located on the ground, using a map and a compass. The winner is the one who finishes the route in the shortest time possible. It is possible to make this competitive against another group or as a single group. You do not have to do it in a running course.

So, how does it work? At the beginning of the route, you get a list of tasks, a check card, and a map. You rely on the compass and on one another, of course. In the end, it is an experience that makes everyone feel great satisfaction and success. There are sites where you can find tracks that have already been built by other people or, with some preparation, you can build one for the whole family.

Find the cache:
The simplest version is to write a few notes with hints where each hint leads to the next location, and the next position will have a note that leads to the next point. The only thing to do is place all the notes in position before starting.

Obstacle race:
You can place obstacles during the race and hand out missions for every obstacle.

Football couples:
Two participants in the game tie one of their legs to each other. They stand side by side, for example, and the right leg of one child is tied to the left leg of the other child. Now, they will need to be totally coordinated with each other when they need to move in any direction.

Leading a blind man:

The participants divide into pairs. Each pair covers the eyes of one of the participants, and the participant with open eyes leads the participant whose eyes are covered. In the next round, the roles change. You can ban speech, you can prohibit contact, you can create obstacle courses, and more. The experiences lead to the opening for many discussions, trust, responsibility, cooperation, sensory deprivation, disabilities, and so on.

Catching hugs:

If two people are hugging, they cannot be caught. So, whoever is "it" tries to catch another participant in the game who isn't being hugged. As soon as a person is caught not being hugged, they are the new "it," and they must find someone who isn't being hugged.

Dancing party:

For this fun activity, you do not even have to leave the house. All you need is to announce a stormy dance party and send everyone to get organized. First of all, you need a good dance floor, so clear the living room of furniture and other obstacles. In the second stage, the shutters and windows are covered, darkening the room and creating an atmosphere. You can bring in a floor lamp or turn on light, but everything else goes.

The next step, and the most important step, is the music. This stage is actually worth doing with the children, and it will make them much more enthusiastic and involved. We recommend that you make a playlist on YouTube or in the iTunes album. You can choose in such a way that each member of the family chooses another song, and that's

225

how everyone is active in the selection. You can repeat the same action until you have a decent playlist. This playlist can be used again and again in many situations. When everything is ready, everyone goes to dress up, like before a class party, in beautiful and comfortable clothes, and then the fun begins. The volume is turned up and everyone dances together.

Summary

You are a small part of people who started and finished this book. It is a sign that your family and people close to you are important to you. It is a sign that you know what is important to you in life and that you are ready to do what you need for your life to be like what you want.

Now is the time to put it into practice. Take this book and implement the same actions in your daily life. Hold it close to you and go over and over it again to sharpen each subject until you feel that you are in control of each of the four elements.

So, what did we do in this book?

Until now, we have talked about the four elements for a long and healthy life and how to assimilate it into the family: body and mind, habits and the environment, nutrition, and exercise.

These four elements support each other in perfect synchronization. Each part of this equation requires the other. Each part has its importance and it holds the entire structure stable and strong.

Each part has an effect on another part. While each part has its own great importance in its own right, each part has an impact on the whole.

I really want to thank you personally for taking the time to read this book. I sincerely hope that I have contributed to your family's health. I truly believe that you can make a significant difference in your life and your family and you have all the capabilities and tools to do it. I wish you years

Made in the USA
Middletown, DE
11 June 2018